The Com Vagus Nerve ~~Exercises~~

Heal, stimulate, and exercise your vagus nerve naturally.
Renew your mind with healing exercises for your body

2-Week Meal Plan

BY
Matthew Rappazzo

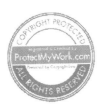

Table of Contents

Introduction

We all know how important it is to stay healthy and fit. But did you know that there is a nerve in your body that could help you achieve this? It's called the vagus nerve, one of the body's most significant nerves. In this book, we'll look at the vagus nerve, its advantages, how to exercise it, and how to stimulate it for optimal health.

So let's get started!

The vagus nerve is quite possibly the biggest nerve in your body, running from the brainstem to the mid-region. It controls digestion, heart rate, and respiration, among other bodily functions. Emotional regulation, inflammation, and immunity are all regulated by it. The vagus nerve is part of the "parasympathetic nervous system" (PNS). This system calms the body and gives it time to rest and digest. Additionally, it is accountable for promoting feelings of well-being and stress management. The vagus nerve is called the "wandering nerve" since it branches throughout the body. This indicates that it is in close proximity to numerous organs in the body, such as the lungs, heart, and digestive system.

The vagus nerve has many advantages, and actuating it can assist with working on general well-being. One of the main benefits of the vagus nerve is its ability to regulate the body's response to stress. The body can relax and lower stress levels by stimulating the vagus nerve. The vagus nerve likewise assumes a part in managing feelings. Anxiety and depression can be reduced by stimulating the vagus nerve. Additionally, it may assist in enhancing mood and well-being.

The vagus nerve is also important for digestion. Stimulating the vagus nerve can help increase stomach acid production and digestion. It can also help to reduce bloating and improve nutrient absorption. Finally, activating the vagus nerve can help to boost the immune system. Stimulating the vagus nerve can help to reduce inflammation and improve immunity.

There are several exercises that can help to activate the vagus nerve. These exercises can help reduce stress and promote relaxation and well-being. Deep breathing is one of the most effective exercises for activating the vagus nerve. Deep breathing is a relaxation method that involves slow breathing through the nose and out through the mouth. Focusing on the breath as it enters and exits the body is required for deep breathing. The vagus nerve may be stimulated through deep breathing, lowering stress levels.

Another exercise for stimulating the vagus nerve is humming. Humming involves taking a deep breath and then humming for a few seconds. This can help to activate the vagus nerve and reduce stress. Gargling is also an effective exercise for stimulating the vagus nerve. The goal of gargling is to make a low humming sound while inhaling and exhaling. Finally, yoga involves stretching and breathing exercises that can help to relax the body and reduce stress.

There are various techniques that can be used to stimulate the vagus nerve. These techniques can reduce stress and promote relaxation. One of the most popular techniques is cold exposure. Cold exposure involves taking a cold shower or bath or immersing the body in cold water. That can help to activate the vagus nerve and reduce stress levels. Another technique for stimulating the vagus nerve is massage. Massage can reduce body tension and increase blood flow. Stress may be reduced, and the vagus nerve may be stimulated. The vagus nerve can also be effectively stimulated with acupuncture.

The practice of acupuncture consists of inserting particular needles into specific body parts. This can help to activate the vagus nerve and reduce stress levels. Finally, yoga can also be used to stimulate the vagus nerve. Yoga involves stretching and breathing exercises that can help to reduce stress and activate the vagus nerve.

This book is intended to be a practical guide that reveals the secrets of the vagus nerve, providing you with an excellent blueprint for transforming your health. You will learn about the different roles of the vagus nerve for general health through step-by-step instructions and helpful advice. You will also learn how to exercise (even for 5 minutes a day) and strengthen your nerve to manage chronic conditions, improve bodily functioning, and conquer mental health issues.

Stimulating the Vagus Nerve for Good Mental Health

The body's superpower is the vagus nerve, which combats the fight-or-flight reaction. By this interaction, you make a solid pressure reaction and become strong. You feel more serene, humane, and clear when you are animated. Your mental and autonomic nervous systems benefit from stimulating the vagus nerve. Emotional control increased connection and improved physical health are all signs of healthy vagal tones. You have greater resilience and are able to overcome adversity and trauma.

The Vagus Nerve: What Is It?

The vagus nerve is a vital and complex part of the body's nervous system. As the longest cranial nerve, the vagus nerve extends throughout the body, connecting the brainstem to various organs and muscles. This is why it is often referred to as the "wandering" nerve.

The word "vagus" is derived from Latin, and it means "wandering." This is fitting, given the vagus nerve's ability to connect and influence many body parts. The vagus nerve is a type of nerve found only in mammals, and it plays a crucial role in the immune system's ability to fight off diseases and the body's inflammation responses.

The vagus nerve has three main functions: motor, parasympathetic, and special sensory. It is responsible for the dorsal and ventral sections of the body and plays a crucial role in regulating various bodily functions such as heart rate, digestion, and immune function.

Overall, the vagus nerve is an essential part of the body's overall health and well-being. By taking care of it and engaging in practices that support its health, you can help to ensure that it is functioning at its best and supporting your overall health and well-being.

When it comes to the body's response to the environment, the vagus nerve plays a crucial role. The front part of the body is called the ventral area, while the back part is called the dorsal area, and both areas of the brain may be involved in the process of evaluating environmental cues for safety or danger, a process called neuroception.

Safety signals activate the ventral area, while danger signals activate the dorsal area. In response to the environment, a person can be in one of three states: mobilization, immobilization, or social engagement. A functioning vagal nerve helps a person respond thoughtfully rather than reacting automatically.

For example, if you encounter a threatening or dangerous situation, your vagus nerve may activate the dorsal area of your brain, prompting you to prepare for fight or flight. On the other hand, if you encounter a situation that feels safe and supportive, your vagus nerve may activate the ventral area of your brain, prompting you to relax and engage socially. Overall, the vagus nerve is essential to the body's ability to navigate and respond to the environment in a healthy and balanced way. By taking care of your vagus nerve and engaging in practices that support its health, you can help ensure that you respond thoughtfully to the world around you.

The vagus nerve plays a crucial role in the body's responses to stress, anxiety, and fear. It carries information from the gut to the brain, which helps the body recover from stressful and fearful situations. This is why we often talk about "gut feelings" when it comes to understanding of our own emotions and reactions. When the brain's sympathetic nervous system detects a threat, it triggers the fight or flight response. This is a natural and necessary response that helps us protect ourselves when we are in danger. In contrast, the parasympathetic nervous system helps a person relax. That thong was activated when danger passed, such as when a person was rescued from oncoming traffic while crossing the street. After the danger has passed, a person may feel content and calm.

However, sometimes the brain may remain in a state of panic, causing a person to feel as though they are still in danger. This can lead to persistent feelings of anxiety and fear, even in the absence of any immediate threat. In these cases, it can be helpful to focus on activating the parasympathetic nervous system, where the vagus nerve plays a role. By engaging in practices stimulating the vagus nerve, such as deep breathing or cold exposure, you can help to activate the parasympathetic nervous system and bring about a sense of calm and relaxation. Additionally, the vagus nerve plays a role in feelings of compassion and empathy, so engaging in activities that promote these emotions can also help manage fear and anxiety. Generally, taking care of your vagus nerve can help you better manage your body's responses to stress and fear.

The vagus nerve, that wondrous messenger of calm, recognizes when we are no longer in danger and helps us to stay serene in times of distress. Its "relax and digest" responses involve low-tone activity in the dorsal area, while the parasympathetic nervous system experiences high-tone activity in that same region when we enter a freeze mode. If we are not emotionally healthy, we may find ourselves stuck in either sympathetic mode (the fight or flight response) or parasympathetic mode. In the parasympathetic system, you find two additional states: rest and digestion, which are vital. This branch can help us feel less vigilant and more at ease.

Techniques such as grounding, mindfulness, and self-biofeedback, such as breathing exercises, can help restore the vagus nerve's ability to regulate itself. The vagal tone, which is related to the body's ability to regulate stress reactions, may be influenced by breathing. Practices such as yoga and meditation may help increase vagal tone, reducing mood swings and anxiety symptoms. Another treatment called vagus nerve stimulation (VNS) involves using a device similar to a pacemaker to stimulate the vagus nerve. This is often done in combination with other treatments, such as therapy and antidepressants. Engaging in activities that stimulate the vagus nerve can help a person practice mindfulness and bring their attention back to themselves.

The vagus nerve is closely connected to the heart, intestines, and voice. When people check in with their true emotions, gain intuitive insight, or discover their inner expressiveness, they activate the vagus nerve. The vagus nerve is activated when their face reflects their true feelings or experiences. When they connect with the rhythms of themselves or the world around them, they activate the vagus nerve. When they speak, shout, or sing, the vagus nerve becomes active, which is one reason why these activities can be so emotionally and cathartically impactful for many people.

How to Stimulate Your Vagus Nerve for Good Mental Health

You can reset your ventral vagus nerve with a few exercises for the vagus nerve. They are as follows: The Fundamental Workout, the Half Salamander Workout, and the Full Salamander Workout.

The Fundamental Workout

- Lie on your back.
- Place your intertwined hands behind the head.
- Keep your head still and look to the right.
- Don't move until you feel you must yawn or deglitch.
- Return to a neutral position with straight eyes.
- Repeat on the opposing side.

The eight sub-occipital muscles and the muscles that move our eyes have a "direct neurological relationship.

The Half-Salamander Workout

- Tilt the head to the right, toward the shoulder, without twisting the head.
- Hold for 30 to 60 seconds.
- After that, put your head and eyes back in neutral.
- Tilt your head to the left towards the shoulder without twisting your head.
- Hold for 30 to 60 seconds.
- Then return to neutral.

If you look in the other direction of the head tilt, the eyes will look right, and the head will be tilted to the left. For between 30 and 60 seconds, both hold their necks.

Full Salamander Workout

- Get on all fours and get down.
- "The head is looking down."
- Allow your left spine to rotate while tilting your head to the left; look to the left without rotating your head; tilt your head to the left.
- Press for 30 to 60 seconds.
- Bring your head and spine to the middle for straightening.
- Repeat on the opposing side.

Additional Methods for Stimulating Your Vagus Nerve Includes:

1. Diaphragmatic breathing exercises: Put the first hand on your chest and the second hand on your stomach. Feel your stomach grow as you breathe in, and your stomach ought to contract as you breathe out. Another name for this is "belly breathing." Your heart rate slows down, which lowers your blood pressure.

2. Connection: A sense of community and belonging improves feelings of safety and security. When you're connected, you feel more positive and calmer.

3. The Dive Reflex Cold exposure: is necessary for the diving reflex to be activated. You can use ice cubes in a zip-loc bag to protect your face or splash cold water on it. The diving reflex calms the body, reduces anger, and increases blood flow to the brain.

4. Gargling, humming, or singing: Don't you find that humming or singing makes you feel better? Your worries are washed away by music. This is because it stimulates your vagus nerve! If you want to feel better, all you must do is sing or spit.

5. Gut bacteria: Beneficial microbes in the gut improve brain function thanks to the vagus nerve activation.

6. Omega-3 fatty acids: These can be found in fish oil or in vegan-friendly sources such as chia seeds, hemp seed oil, flaxseed, and nuts.

7. Meditation and mindfulness: Loving-kindness meditation can improve vagal tone. Mindfulness practices, in general, stimulate the vagus nerve. Being present helps to ground a person.

8. Yoga: This practice activates the parasympathetic nervous system, which can improve digestion, blood flow, and other functions.

9. ASMR is a sensation characterized by a tingling sensation that starts from the head and runs down the back. It is often triggered by specific sounds, such as tapping, scraping, or whispering, and is thought to help calm the nervous system. Some people find ASMR helpful in relieving stress or promoting relaxation

10. Chanting "OM" is a practice that is believed to stimulate the vagus nerve and promote relaxation. It is commonly used in yoga, meditation, and various spiritual traditions, such as

Buddhism and Hinduism. Research has shown that chanting "OM" can help increase feelings of relaxation and promote a sense of inner peace. Whether used as a spiritual practice or simply as a relaxation technique, chanting "OM" can effectively promote relaxation and stress reduction.

11. Using positive self-talk can help stimulate the vagus nerve and improve your overall well-being. Even when you feel afraid, acknowledging your courage and speaking positively can help boost your confidence and encourage you to act. Regularly practicing affirmations can be a powerful way to support a healthy vagal tone and improve your overall sense of self. Using positive self-talk, you can tap into the power of the vagus nerve to enhance your overall well-being and become your best self.

How the Vagus Nerve Improves Your Well-Being Positively

The circulatory system, digestive system, reproductive system, and numerous other organs are all connected to the vagus nerve. It receives readings from each and relays brain-derived information, analogous to a neural superhighway. It is the largest nerve of the body.

The vagus nerve is present in virtually every part of your internal organs. It establishes a novel and intriguing connection between the genitals and the brain. The vagus nerve, which is a neuronal highway that runs the length of our bodies, enables many spinal cord injury patients to experience sexual pleasure. Stimulating the vagus nerve and increasing "vagal tone" have been shown to improve mental and physical well-being.

It has the potential to enhance everything, including longevity and appearance. "The future of medicine" is given to the vagus nerve, also known as "the self-care nerve." It may have the solution to a surprising number of current diseases. Anyone worried about their health needs to learn how to use its powers.

The human nervous system is made up of several interconnected parts, including the autonomic nervous system (ANS). The ANS is responsible for regulating functions that occur automatically in the body, such as heart rate, sweating, blood pressure, digestion, and breathing. These functions are not under conscious control, and the ANS plays a crucial role in maintaining homeostasis within the body. The vagus nerve is an important part of the ANS and is involved in regulating many of these autonomic functions.

The ANS is made up of three main components:

The Sympathetic Nervous System (SNS), the Parasympathetic Nervous System (PNS), and the Enteric Nervous System (ENS) (ENS) are all parts of the autonomic nervous system.

The "fight or flight" response is under the control of the SNS. The SNS controls our body's innate response to danger. It speeds up the heart, makes the lungs bigger, and moves blood from organs to muscles. The body gets a lot of oxygen from this, and adrenaline and cortisol are released.

Even though digestion has its distinct reflex activity, there is a connection between the ENS and the function of the intestines. It makes it easier to communicate with the brain and nervous system.

The PNS manages the "rest and digest" mechanism. By slowing down the heart and breathing, it relaxes the body. It moves the body's resources to important organs, allowing more independent processes like digestion to work fully. The vagus nerve is a crucial channel through which various systems communicate. It seems to be the "central switchboard" for the ANS.

Fight or Flight versus Rest and Digestion

The sympathetic nervous system (SNS) is responsible for activating the body's "fight or flight" response in emergencies. This response is designed to temporarily boost energy and strength, allowing a person to fight or escape a potentially dangerous situation. However, the SNS is not meant to be active for long periods of time and should be turned off once the emergency has passed.

To produce a temporary boost of energy and strength, the SNS takes resources away from the other autonomous systems, making the muscles stronger and the senses more alert. The parasympathetic nervous system (PNS) is a counterbalance to the SNS, helping to regulate and inhibit the SNS when it is not needed.

It is not healthy to spend long periods of time in a state of "fight or flight," as this can have negative effects on the body's organs. Unfortunately, modern stressors often involve prolonged mental or emotional strain periods, which can trigger the sympathetic nervous system (SNS) and cause a prolonged "fight or flight" response.

It is necessary to stimulate the vagus nerve and activate the parasympathetic nervous system (PNS) to return the body to a state of normal resting and digestion. This helps to counterbalance the SNS and restore the body's normal resting state.

Stimulating the vagus nerve can help activate the parasympathetic nervous system (PNS), which has a few beneficial effects on the body. For example, the vagus nerve increases the production of stomach acid and digestive enzymes. These enzymes improve your digestion and help ensure that nutrients are absorbed properly and for a long time. In addition, stimulating the vagus nerve can help reduce the pulse and support the proper functioning of the immune system. The production of hormones and enzymes, such as oxytocin and acetylcholine, can also be improved, which can positively affect mental and physical health.

But that's not the end of it.

Microbiome readings can be taken by the vagus nerve, according to research. Then eliciting responses depending on the findings. Additionally, it will activate anxiogenic and anxiolytic effects in response to specific stimuli. Here, we see the significant state of mind adjusting capability of vagal nerve enactment.

There is even some evidence to suggest that controlling inflammatory responses is made possible by learning how to manage the vagus nerve. This effectively prevents the breakdown of cells, reducing the signs of aging. Compared to the medications that are frequently harmful, this is a far superior alternative. By the anti-inflammatory strategy, the vagus nerve can help the body's latent stem cells. This infers that the vagus nerve could decrease cell debasement at any point and invigorate some cell recovery.

The vagal tone refers to the strength, rate, and effectiveness of the vagus nerve in activating the parasympathetic nervous system. It can be measured using an electrocardiogram (ECG), which looks at the difference in heart rate between inhaling and exhaling. A more significant difference indicates a higher vagal tone.

Higher vagal tone is linked to better control of blood glucose levels, which can reduce the risk of conditions such as diabetes, stroke, and cardiovascular disease. Increasing vagal tone can help improve overall health and well-being. Among other things, the low vagal tone has been linked to chronic inflammation, increased stress, and cardiovascular problems. Practicing vagus nerve stimulation can improve vagal tone. There are a few strategies for achieving this, some more intrusive than others. Implantation of a Vagal Nerve Stimulator (VNS) has been used to treat epilepsy and acute migraines since 1997.

Patients typically report improvements in their mental and physical health due to this treatment, which electrically stimulates the nerve. Additionally, there is a significant decrease in migraines and/or seizures. Using a VNS to treat depression, bipolar disorder, and morbid obesity is also well-established.

Vagal Nerve Stimulation Using Less Invasive Treatments

These less invasive treatments can also be used to stimulate the nerve, though the effects are not as dramatic. For instance, it has been demonstrated that carotid sinus massage can slow the heart rate and prevent certain kinds of seizures. Certain yoga techniques can send psychological information back to the brain through the vagus nerve.

Similar to how psychological cues can elicit a bodily "fight or flight" response, physical information can influence a psychological response. The vagus nerve is used to transmit this physical data. You can recreate quiet side effects by utilizing yogic breathing and smooth development. The vagus nerve is stimulated, and this indicates to the brain that everything is fine. Consequently, the mind allows stress to escape.

Hawing and humming

Auditory vibrations can stimulate the vagus nerve. It has been demonstrated that humming and rhythmic chanting are known meditative techniques that stimulate the vagus nerve. Ideally heard through headphones in both ears, softly articulated noises elicit a parasympathetic vagus nerve response.

Exercises for Vagal Tone

One of the most effective non-invasive ways to improve vagal tone is to practice meditative self-care techniques.

The following are some concepts:

- Humming, along with practices such as yogic or meditative breathing and singing, can have a positive impact on the vagus nerve. To get the most benefit, try combining humming with deep, slow inhalations and exhalations through the nose. Focus on how your ribs, throat, mouth, and skull vibrate as you hum and continue until you feel completely relaxed. Other practices that may be helpful for stimulating the vagus nerve include gargling and participating in communal singing, choruses, or prayer.

- Submerging your face in cold water for 30 to 60 seconds can stimulate the vagus nerve and help lower a high heart rate. This activates the "dive reflex," which causes the vagus nerve to signal the heart to slow down to conserve oxygen. The dive reflex is a powerful way to stimulate the vagus nerve and can have several positive effects, including reducing anxiety, stress, and body-wide inflammation. Another effective method for stimulating the vagus nerve is to rub ice from the scalp to the lips using a large zip-lock bag.

- Meditation is an effective way to stimulate the vagus nerve and improve overall well-being. There are many different types of meditation practices to choose from, and what works best for one person may not be the best fit for another. It may take some trial and error to find a meditation practice that works for you, but with regular practice, you can improve your vagal tone and experience the benefits of meditation.

Vagus Nerve Exercise

You might not realize it, but you have a relaxation button in your back pocket. It is referred to as the vagus nerve. The parasympathetic nervous system (PNS) is triggered by the vagus nerve, which connects the body and the brain. The two parts of the sensory system are the thoughtful sensory system, associated with the "survival" response, and the parasympathetic sensory system, related to "rest and review."

Obviously, your back pocket does not actually contain the vagus nerve, which originates in the brainstem and runs down the neck to the abdomen. Its primary functions are regulating your heart rate, breathing rate, and digestion. When activated, it reduces your body's physiological response to stress, making you feel more at ease. So, what's the good news? You can activate your vagus nerve by performing specific activities.

Trying to avoid stress is a futile game. Because stress is so common, how you deal with it has the greatest impact on your overall well-being. Vagus nerve stimulation can thus be used as a relaxation therapy whenever you need to unwind.

There are numerous techniques to activate this nerve that can be enjoyable, soothing, or integrated into your everyday routine. You can choose the activities that make you happy rather than having to participate in them all. You can select the ones that you need right now, or that speak to you. The vagus nerve exercises below should be done for five minutes daily.

1. SKY Yoga

Sudarshan Kriya, or SKY yoga as it is commonly known, is a powerful technique that harnesses the power of the breath to bring about a sense of calm and clarity in the mind. This focused breathing practice has been shown to have some physical and mental benefits.

For starters, it has been found to help reduce heart rate and blood pressure, leading to a more relaxed and centered state of being. This can help to improve focus and concentration, making it an excellent tool for anyone looking to improve their productivity and focus.

In addition to its physical benefits, SKY yoga has also been shown to impact mental health positively. Studies have found that it may be particularly effective in reducing sadness and anxiety in individuals who do not respond well to traditional medications. This makes it a valuable tool for those seeking relief from these common mental health issues.

Finally, SKY yoga has been found to improve the quality of one's sleep, helping individuals to get a more restful night's rest. All in all, Sudarshan Kriya is a highly effective and transformative practice that has the potential to enhance both physical and mental well-being."

"If you're looking to try Sudarshan Kriya yoga, or SKY yoga as it is commonly known, it's best to start by finding a class or instructor who can guide you through the practice. A typical SKY yoga class will last for about 45 minutes and will include three different breathing exercises, each performed at a different speed.

First, find a comfortable seat with your legs crossed and your body upright. You may want to close your eyes slightly to help focus your attention inward. Take a deep breath in and exhale while making the sound "om." This simple act of vocalizing creates vibrations in your core and may stimulate the vagus nerve, which regulates the body's stress response.

After focusing on the vibration behind your belly button for a moment, you may want to pause to observe any sensations, thoughts, emotions, or images that arise. You are free to repeat this process three times or as many times as you feel comfortable.

If the "om" sound doesn't resonate with you, you can try using the sound "voo" or other techniques such as humming or vocal gargling to achieve a similar effect. Remember, the vagus nerve connects the muscles in the back of the throat, so any activity that engages these muscles has the potential to stimulate the vagus nerve and promote relaxation.

Overall, SKY yoga is a simple yet powerful practice that can help to reduce stress, enhance focus, and promote a sense of calm and well-being. Give it a try and see how it works for you!"

2. Box Breathing

Box breathing, also known as square breathing or four-square breathing, is a simple yet powerful technique that can help to regulate the body's fight or flight response. When we experience stress or danger, our bodies naturally respond by increasing heart rate and respiration to prepare us to take action.

However, this response can sometimes become overactive, leading to feelings of anxiety and panic. That's where box breathing comes in. By taking longer, deeper, and more mindful breaths, we can signal to the brain that we are safe, which can help to balance activity in the sympathetic and parasympathetic nervous systems and reduce anxiety.

To practice box breathing, find a comfortable seated position and close your eyes if you like. Begin by taking a deep inhalation through the nose, counting to four as you do so. Hold the breath for another four counts, then exhale slowly through the nose for another four counts.

Finally, hold your breath for the final four counts before starting the cycle again. Repeat this process for a total of five minutes, focusing on the sensation of the breath as it moves in and out of the body. With regular practice, box breathing can help to reduce stress and promote a sense of calm and well-being.

Give it a try and see how it works for you!" Here is the process for box breathing:
- Start by gradually releasing all of your lungs' air.
- Inhale slowly while counting down to four.
- For four counts, hold your breath.
- Take a slow exhale for four more counts.
- Hold your breath for a further four counts before inhaling to complete the cycle and count to four.
- Three to five more times, repeat.

3. The cold exposure

If you want to stimulate the vagus nerve to reduce stress, you may consider cold exposure. The shock of the cold activates the sympathetic nervous system, which can help lower the heart rate and redirect blood flow to the brain. This can have a calming effect on the body and mind, making it a helpful tool for those feeling anxious, distressed, or overwhelmed.

There are several different ways you can incorporate cold exposure into your routine. One option is to place a cold compress on your upper chest or face or to take a cold shower. Alternatively, you can end your shower with cold water for the last two to five minutes. The neck area is particularly effective for cold stimulation, so you may want to focus on this area if you're looking for a targeted effect.

Keep in mind that cold exposure can be invigorating, so it's important to first listen to your body and take it slowly. Start with a shorter duration of cold exposure and gradually increase the time as you become more comfortable. With regular practice, you may find that cold exposure has a noticeable calming effect on your body and mind. Give it a try and see how it works for you!

4. Physical activity

Physical activity is an excellent way to tone the vagus nerve, especially exercises that increase your heart rate. In fact, after a cycling session or other high-intensity workout, you may notice that the vagus nerve is more activated, leading to a sense of calm and relaxation. Some of the best forms of exercise for the vagus nerve include walking, weightlifting, swimming, and Pilates cardio, all of which challenge your ability to control your breathing. These activities can help to calm the vagus nerve by making your body work hard, which can positively impact your mental and physical well-being.

However, it's important to be mindful of your limits and avoid overtraining, as strenuous workouts such as high-intensity interval training (HIIT) can tire the vagus nerve. To protect your vagus nerve while exercising, be sure to include cool-downs and breathing exercises in your routine and to take rest days consistently. Overall, regular physical activity is a great way to tone the vagus nerve and promote a sense of calm and well-being. Find an activity you enjoy and make it a regular part of your routine for the best results.

5. Diaphragmatic breathing techniques

Diaphragmatic breathing techniques, such as the three-part breath, can help lower stress hormone cortisol levels. To practice the three-part breath, follow these steps:

- If you're looking to strengthen your vagus nerve and promote relaxation, you may want to try a simple breathing exercise called diaphragmatic breathing. This technique involves focusing on the movement of the breath as it flows in and out of the body and can be an effective way to reduce stress and promote a sense of calm.
- To practice diaphragmatic breathing, start by finding a comfortable seated or lying position. Slowly inhale through your nose (your stomach will expand, and your rib cage will fill). Finally, the air will enter your upper chest.
- After 5 seconds, slowly exhale from the chest, then the rib cage, and finally the belly. After another 5 seconds, repeat the exercise another three times. You can do this exercise anytime, anywhere, and it can be especially helpful when you're feeling anxious or stressed.

- Remember to keep your focus on the sensation of the breath as it moves in and out of the body. With regular practice, diaphragmatic breathing can help to strengthen the vagus nerve and promote a sense of calm and well-being. Give it a try and see how it works for you!"

Deep breathing can help to relax the body and mind and may be helpful in reducing stress and anxiety.

6. Repeat a specific sequence

To help relax and release tension throughout the day, it can be helpful to reset the vagus nerve every morning by following a specific sequence. One such sequence involves pressing inward and to the right with your right index and middle fingers above your navel, then using the same two fingers to press to the left and above your navel. This process can help restore the function of the vagus nerve and promote a sense of calm and relaxation. You can repeat this sequence as needed throughout the day to help maintain a sense of balance and well-being.

- Here's a great way to reduce stress through vagus nerve stimulation: with your fingertips, massage the scalp from the nape of the neck to the forehead, applying gentle pressure.
- Then, press locations just above your navel with one hand while pressing the top of your head with the other.
- Repeat this sequence three times, then take a deep breath. If done correctly, you should feel your jaw relax, your neck loosens, and your shoulders move away from your ears. Your breath should also become deeper. You can try the technique again if you don't notice any results.

7. Fear tap

The "fear tap" method is designed to reduce irrational fear, calm the fight-or-flight response, and stabilize the mind. Left hand with palm facing downwards. Then, with the right-hand, press on the back of your left hand halfway between the wrist and fingers, between the ring and pinkie fingers, for about 30 seconds.

While doing so, inhale with your nose and exhale with your mouth. This technique can be repeated as needed to help reduce stress and anxiety.

8. The cat/cow stretch

The cat/cow stretch is a useful yoga asana for stimulating the vagus nerve. Sit on the edge of the chair and, while exhaling, bring your chin to your chest by bending your back. On the inhale, open your spine, bring your heart forward, and pull your shoulder blades back. Take a deep breath in and out, rounding your back and contracting your core. This stretch can be repeated several times to help relax the body and mind.

9. Hands on the forehead

To reduce reactivity, put your hands on your forehead, one on top of the other. This will create a position as if you are checking for a fever. By breathing into your lower belly for 30 seconds with your eyes closed, you can draw blood up to the forebrain, which can help decrease reactivity. This process can help to relax the body and mind and may be helpful in reducing stress.

10. Scan the entire body

After assessing your level of reactivity, you can conduct a second brief scan of your entire body to help prepare for the day. From head to toe, keep your eyes closed. So, your body should be in a specific state, free from reactivity, to function optimally and fully.

It is important to clear stress reactivity in the morning, as this is when your body processes the stresses of the day. To do this, you can try performing the following scan for ten seconds: sit or stand upright with your feet parallel to the ground and your arms at your sides, then take a deep breath in. This can help to relax the body and mind and prepare you for the day ahead.

11. A long exhale

For mind and body relaxation, taking a long exhale is essential.

Your vagus nerve will be stimulated by simply exhaling more deeply. Deep, slow breathing for two minutes increased activity in the vagus nerve, which led to a longer interval between each heartbeat. You might be able to make better choices as a result!

According to careful analysis, broadening the breathed-out breath conveys a correspondence to the cerebrum through the vagus nerve that your body might calm down, bringing about both physical and mental rest, and may try and incite rest.

While lying down, take four counts of inhalation and four counts of exhalation. After inhaling for four seconds and exhaling for five, the ratio of inhalations to exhalations will gradually increase to four to eight, or 1:2. It might be so effective that you won't even notice you're sleeping!

12. Stretch your neck

Stretch your neck to tone your vagus muscles.

The sternocleidomastoid muscle, which runs down the side of your neck, is also strained due to this. Migraine sufferers frequently hold tension in this region. Simply incline your head and right ear gently toward your right shoulder while placing your right hand on top of your head. Gaze upward for 30 seconds, then recurrent on the opposite side.

13. Torso stretching

The vagus nerve is stimulated by torso stretching.

By moving the rib cage and calming the nervous system, this Yoga U exercise stimulates the vagus nerve in the torso. Now, turn around. Place your abandoned hand and your right hand outwardly of your left leg. Over your left shoulder, look. Lengthen your spine on the inhale and deepen the twist on the exhale. Next, switch sides.

14. Ear massages can alleviate headaches.

The vagus nerve is linked to the upper part of the ear. Tension can influence this area, although this may appear to be a minor movement. When you tone the vagus nerve, which is also connected to the throat and chest, your neck may relax, making breathing easier through the nose.

Over the ridge of your ear canal, gently slide one finger in moderate circles. On the opposing side, respond. Move the ear up and down as you pull it away from the skull. This could assist with temporomandibular joint agony and pressure migraines. Repeat on the opposite side, moving your finger up and down over the area behind the ear. Through the vagus nerve, you are sending messages of relaxation to the brain while massaging the area.

15. Gargling and singing

Several activities that involve manipulating the vocal cords can physically stimulate the vagus nerve. These include gargling and singing.

•   To try gargling, rinse your mouth with water after brushing your teeth in the morning and at night, and then set a timer for 30 seconds to one minute. You can also stimulate the vagus nerve by singing along to your favorite songs, regardless of your vocal ability.

•   Chanting the "om" sound, as is done in yoga, is another activity that can stimulate the vagus nerve through physical means. These activities may trigger the vagus nerve by causing physical vibrations in the vocal cords. To try this technique, sit quietly and chant a long "om." You should be able to feel the vibrations in your ears, and this vibration will connect to the vagus nerve. Chanting "om" can help deactivate the amygdala, a part of the brain's limbic system involved in emotional and stress responses.

•   Laughing is another activity that can stimulate the vagus nerve. To get this benefit, you can watch a funny movie or TV show and laugh out loud at the amusing parts or spend time with a friend who loves slapstick humor.

16. Emotions and thoughts

In addition to physically activating the vagus nerve through breathing exercises and cold exposure, you can also stimulate the nerve through your emotions and thoughts. By evoking an emotional response that is beneficial for the vagus nerve, you can help the parasympathetic nervous system relax. This suggests that it is possible to influence the vagus nerve through psychological and physical means.

- Writing down three things you are grateful for before going to bed or when you wake up, whether they are large or small, can help to stimulate the parasympathetic nervous system (PNS). This practice can be done daily, weekly, or at any frequency that works best for you.

- Deep inhalation, such as the box breathing or square breathing exercise, which involves holding the breath for a count of four on the exhale and four on the exhale, can also help activate the PNS. By taking slow, deep breaths, your body may perceive that you are not in danger and respond by activating the PNS. As needed, you can repeat the exercise.

- Meditation and other "contemplative activities", such as yoga, have been shown to promote a sense of peace and relaxation, in part, by activating the vagus nerve. Meditation can take many forms and does not have to be lengthy to be effective. For five minutes, you can try using a guided meditation app like Headspace, Calm, or Insight Timer.

- Additionally, engaging in activities that bring positive emotions, such as enjoying a sunset, spending time in nature, looking at beautiful pictures, or playing with pets, can also increase vagal tone and contribute to good physical health. These activities may vary from person to person in terms of what elicits positive emotions.

17. Increased Salivation

The mind becomes calmer and more relaxed the easier it is to salivate. Your body enters parasympathetic mode when the mouth produces an excessive amount of saliva. This causes stimulation of the Vagus Nerve. Try sitting in a chair and picturing a juicy lemon to make yourself salivate more. Simply relaxing yourself will make more saliva secreted. But, if salivation does not increase, put some water in your mouth and keep your tongue relaxed. Your hands, feet, hips, neck, and brain will all relax as you relax even more. Hold this sensation for as long as possible by taking a deep breath.

18. Music

Music has the power to move us, bring us joy, and tap into our feelings. There are a lot of contradictory studies on how music affects the vagus nerve. Your inner ear is where your vagus nerve connects to your vocal cords and the muscles at the back of your throat.

19. Vergence

Practicing vergence is the first step in activating your Vagus nerve. The vergence therapy technique is a straightforward strategy for calming your body and activating your vagus nerve. How does Vergence aid in relaxation and anxiety reduction? The six muscles holding your eyes in place are called extraocular muscles, or EOMs. Your oculocardiac reflex (OCR) originates in extraocular muscles composed of numerous nerve endings. A quick way to unwind is to use the oculocardiac reflex. You are stimulating your OCR and, as a result, your vagus nerve when you switch your focus between two close and far objects.

Using Vergence Therapy:
- "Get your pen out!"
- Close your eyes for three seconds while holding a pen or your finger six inches in front of you.
- Focus your attention for three seconds on a point about 10 feet away through the pen.

- Return your focus to the pen (close point) for three seconds.
- Move your attention away from the pen for approximately two to three minutes.
- You can set a timer on your phone to help you keep track of time!

20. Plunge Reaction in Mammalian

The Mammalian Plunge Reaction is the second component to enact your Vagus nerve. When submerged in cold water, the mammalian diving reflex of humans quickly kicks in. The dive reaction will slow your heart rate and breathing, which will help calm you down and lessen your panic.

- Fill half of a basin with ice-cold water.
- Immerse your head in the bowl for fifteen seconds.
- A very cool shower is another chance.

21. The trapezius twist

Also known as the vagus nerve hack is a great exercise to perform immediately after sitting for an extended period. If you are having trouble maintaining your posture or if you feel like your head is just tipping forward, the trapezius twist will help you get your muscles working. Brain activity activates muscles. Compare your forward head before and after the workout to see the difference.

For this exercise, hug yourself and rotate your pelvis to the left and right 5 times. Then raise your arms to chest height and turn another 5 times. Then proceed to the chest line for five seconds. Finally, elevate your shoulders for five seconds. Check your forward head posture once more after you finish.

22. The Egyptian sphinx

It is another powerful vagus nerve hack. The sphinx can increase blood flow to the brainstem and activate the vagus nerve, which can improve the cervical range of motion. To begin this exercise, prop yourself up to your elbows while lying on your stomach. Start with your head centered, lift your pubic bone off the ground gently, spin to the left for 30 seconds, and then repeat. After that, move to the right for 30 seconds before returning to the center.

After the exercise, you will see that your range of motion will improve. On the off chance that it feels improved, it was intended to unwind or invigorate cranial nerve XI, the assistant nerve. The SCM and trapezius muscles will both be relaxed as a result. If it did not, it suggests that a different cranial nerve is the source of the issue. Just keep in mind that there are a variety of exercises that might work better for you.

We all once occupied this developmental position as infants. When we prop ourselves up on our forearms, our posture changes. Additionally, it has the highest reflexive stability. Working and exercising from this stance, movement, and postures is excellent. This is a great exercise to try if you frequently suffer from migraines or a stiff neck.

23. Pelvic Floor Unwinding

Pelvic floor delivery and unwinding is another magnificent vagus nerve hack because the vagus nerve is also connected to the nervous system in the gastrointestinal tract and pelvis. Since we typically keep so much stress here, the pelvic floor is interesting. This is additionally where we will quite often keep our feelings.

Sitting on a ball and working on the muscles in the pelvic floor can produce this effective relaxation response. To target the front of the pelvic floor, the ball is placed behind the pubic bone, and to target the back of the pelvic floor, it is placed right inside the buttocks. Sitting on the ball, relax as you breathe through your diaphragm.

There are numerous variations of this excellent relaxation technique. However, all you need to do is adopt a posture that allows you to inhale the pelvic floor and is extremely comfortable for you. The pelvic outlet is opened, and the pelvic floor is relaxed when you inhale.

To instigate that unwinding response, you're opening the pelvic outlet and breathing in into the foundation of the pelvic floor. From a chakra perspective, it's good to address this because the pelvic floor has one of the most fascinating connections to the vagus nerve. It is a place where you can keep your emotions in check and clench your teeth.

24. Neck Release

To perform this exercise correctly:
1. Place a tennis ball under your ear.
2. Gently squeeze the ball and twist it around the entire neck.
3. Be gentle in the center of the neck, where the pharynx, larynx, and esophagus are.

You can help by moving your head in the opposite direction.

So, what are some of the things you might feel after completing this exercise?

- Your face and neck may feel significantly more relaxed or softened.
- You may experience a sigh, swallow, or yawn, indicating nervous system relaxation.

- You may experience facial warmth.
- You could notice that you can see, hear, or talk more clearly. This is due to vagus nerve stimulation and activation of other facial and cranial nerves.

Carry the ball with you at all times, and you can do these exercises whenever you want, even if you are away from home. It could return you to a parasympathetic state, a state of social involvement in which you are connected, mindful, and joyful.

25. Auricular Ear Release

Under the ridge in your ear, place your finger. You ought to think about pressing backward. Use your finger to make slow, minute circles. Although it may feel different from side to side, there should be no pain or discomfort. A yawn, swallow, or sigh might come from this. That indicates that the nervous system has relaxed. Most likely, you should feel at ease.

The second way would be to come down nearly as if you were trying to insert your finger into the eardrum. Perform slow, smooth circles while gently pressing backward toward the back of your head. This could be done for one minute or for as long as you feel it is beneficial and comfortable.

The third approach involves inserting your finger behind your ear on the skin. You will gently draw the skin up and over the tissue, pushing it in the direction of your head. This is referred to as a myofascial release. Hold the position until you feel a release. This may cause your finger to move more easily and your skin to feel more elastic. It may also cause a relaxing reaction. You can hold this for one minute or longer if it is beneficial to you.

The final method is to pull down the ear lobe gently. Because this is a craniosacral method, it may help with dizziness, headaches, and other neurological issues. This is effective for various reasons, not just activating the vagus nerve.

After finishing one side, turn to the other and review to see whether it feels more elastic and less irritating. The benefit of these vagus nerve hacks is that they give you power over your neural system. You may incorporate these into your daily routine because they just take seconds to minutes to complete. This will help you return to a state of rest and digestion, as well as a condition of social interaction in which you can be joyous, attentive, grounded, and compassionate.

26. Valsalva Maneuver

The Valsalva maneuver is beneficial for anyone with supraventricular tachycardia (SVT) or an increased heart rate. In essence, it will lower the heart rate and induce calm.

- Inhale normally, squeeze your nostrils, and exhale slowly.
- Hold for ten seconds. You're exhaling through your nose while compressing your nasal valves, causing pressure in your chest.

First, assess your feelings, and then repeat this process multiple times. It should result in a slower heartbeat and a relaxing reaction. Taking your pulse before and after the maneuver is a wonderful way to see if it has dropped your heart rate. You can utilize either your radial or carotid pulse, whichever is more convenient for you. Just make sure not to take your pulse with your thumb. The Valsalva maneuver can be a very beneficial addition to your life and health.

27. Hand Reflexology

Our vagus nerve accounts for 80% of our parasympathetic nervous system; therefore, it can help with heart rate, digestion, and overall calm.

Reflexology is founded on the Chinese medical concept of Qi, or vital energy. Qi circulates differently through our bodies, but when we are stressed, it tends to become obstructed, and it can become blocked in certain places of the body. Different regions of our bodies are associated with different reflexology or pressure points in Chinese medicine. For example, the vagus nerve point in your hand is located just inside the pinky. This is fantastic because it is easily available throughout the day.

- Apply pressure to the inside of your fifth finger, the pinky. Begin by applying sustained pressure for 30 to 60 seconds.
- Then, while applying pressure to the skin, draw little circles in that area.
- Finally, make feather-light strokes back and forth. This can be done for 30 to 60 seconds.

When you do these exercises, you will feel more relaxed. The signs can be a yawn, a sigh, a swallow, or just a sense of serenity.

Like all of the other hacks we've discussed so far, this is a simple technique for managing your nervous system during the day. When you're stressed, you can easily use one of these three approaches, or all three, to induce a relaxation reaction. If you found this helpful, please incorporate it into your daily routine.

28. Breathing before Eating

Stimulation of the paradigmatic nervous system through breathing can improve digestion. Every day, we breathe 20,000 to 25,000 times. Because the esophagus runs through the diaphragm, it can get constricted, resulting in symptoms such as acid reflux.

We aim to improve the bidirectional connection between our stomach and brain because 80% of afferent information travels from the gut to the brain. We accomplish this by breathing diaphragmatically.

This implies that when you inhale, your belly button moves toward your spine, and when you exhale, your belly button moves away from your spine. This is why breathing using the neck and shoulder muscles is best, without expanding the rib cage.

Simply taking 3-10 diaphragmatic breaths before eating will greatly aid digestion.

29. Acupuncture

Acupuncture is an ancient medical treatment that is thought to balance the flow of chi or qi, the body's vital energy. Acupuncture works by enhancing vagal tone, which is one of the evidence-based ways it works. The vagus nerve is stimulated by traditional acupuncture sites, particularly those in the ear, just as it does in reflexology. What's more, in both healthy people and heart patients, reflexology stimulates the vagus nerve.

30. Aromatherapy

Aromatherapy is the therapeutic application of essential oils and other aromatic substances to improve physical or mental well-being. Relaxing essential scents like lavender and bergamot improve heart rate variability. Surprisingly, some studies suggest that essential oils are not required. Simply inhaling a pleasant aroma or recalling joyful memories might activate the parasympathetic nervous system.

Quick Exercises to Do When You Don't Have Time

Despite the numerous advantages and conveniences offered by modern technology, one major drawback remains: Many of us sit at a desk for at least eight hours a day, five days a week, most of the year.

Unfortunately, the same thing that can keep us busy, make us money, and be good employees for our company can also hurt our health, possibly for good. Weight gain, coronary illness, diabetes, hypertension, and other constant ailments can be ascribed to inordinate sitting.

One alarming study found that sitting all day increases mortality risk by 40%. We don't say that your job will kill you, but it's a good idea to take some simple measures to improve your health at work. An excellent place to begin is simply moving your body more frequently at work. If you work from home and want to exercise with your team virtually, you might want to organize a work-related online fitness class.

You can participate more actively at work. Also, improving your health and well-being at work doesn't require much effort. I've compiled a list of easy desk-friendly activities that will help you combat the negative effects of sitting all day to get you started. These activities include little ventures and will assist you with staying in shape and vivacious during the normal business day.

That's all there is to it: You'll feel better the more you move. Therefore, the next time you experience the sensation that your back is firmly fixed to your desk chair, try a few, all of them, or all of them. They will get your blood flowing, help you build strength, reduce stiffness and injury, and more.

Make your muscles feel great by combining them with branded fitness gear and a few flexibility exercises!

1. Start-up Meeting

The start-up meeting prepares the department for a good day. It's likewise a decent chance to extend your muscles in anticipation of your work environment exercise.

Start with the neck and work your direction down.

- Alternate sides, tilt your head toward your neck, and stretch your shoulders to improve strength and flexibility.
- Roll shoulders in a circular motion forward, then backward.
- Continue 10 times.

Stretch your wrists before working at a computer to get ready. Stretch your arm out.
- With the second hand, pull the fingers down.
- Keep it there for 5 seconds.
- After that, pull upward with your fingers.
- Keep it there for 5 seconds.
- Alternate every 3 times.

If you stretch your calves and ankles, you might feel less tired and lethargic in your legs.

- "Keep one leg straight and raise the other foot off the ground."
- Flex your ankle with your toes pointing upward.
- Point your toes downward while extending your ankle.
- "Ten times with the other leg, repeat."
- Then, using your toes, move one foot clockwise and then counterclockwise to form a circle.
- Pull out your shoes.

2. Exercise with a copier

While you are waiting for copies to be made, you can use the time to do some leg exercises to improve your strength and tone. Some simple leg lifts and swings, which use your body weight and the muscles in your legs, can be done while standing near the copier for balance. Just be mindful of your surroundings and stop the exercise if someone approaches.

To do leg lifts and swings:
- Stand with the left leg straight and lift the right leg to the side or back
- Slowly lower the left leg
- Switch sides
- Bend your left knee
- Swing your leg forward and back 10 times
- Repeat with the right leg.

To do glute kicks:

- Stand with one leg straight and kick your buttocks with the heel of the opposite leg
- Repeat from 12 to 15 times with the two legs.

To do calf raises:
- Stand and lift heels off the ground, then slowly lowering them
- Repeat from 12 to 15 times

3. Workout on the desk

While you read a document, you are also working on strengthening your core and relieving tired leg muscles.
- Place your feet flat on the ground at the start.
- Take a seated position at your desk.
- Get your abdominal muscles to contract.
- Reach the level of your hip with one leg.
- Ten seconds must be spent in that position.
- Slowly lower your leg.
- Rehash multiple times more.

4. Squats in a chair

Chair squats are an excellent exercise for building muscle.
Keep your back straight.
- To do some leg toning exercises:
- Pretend to sit down by lowering your chair one inch and hold that position for ten seconds, then stand up.
- Keep your legs straight and cross one over the other.
- Lift them off the ground and apply pressure with the top leg while resisting with the bottom leg.
- Continue until you feel tired, then switch and use the opposite legs.

5. To stay visible and healthy at work:

- Visit coworkers instead of sending emails to keep your projects and body moving
- Drink plenty of water, as it can help you lose weight, and the more you use the bathroom, the more calories you'll burn
- Go to a bathroom that is further away from your workstation to burn more calories and potentially meet new people
- Walk quickly instead of running to raise your pulse and give the impression of being busy
- Take the stairs instead of the elevator whenever possible, and try using them two at a time for a better workout

6. Abdominal exercises that can be done while sitting in an office chair

Use an exercise ball as an office chair for all-day abdominal training and strengthening, and engage your abs to stay in place while sitting on it.

It helps alleviate lower back pain, strengthens core muscles, and improves balance. Some even claim that it aids in concentration. Find your center of gravity by sitting on the ball. Increase your navel. Step your shoulders back (no slumping).

Place your feet shoulder-width apart. It's difficult to sit on an activity ball. Most likely, you should begin at home to determine your endurance.

7. Bottom-Line Movers

In addition to helping your own bottom line, you can also help the bottom line of your business. Attempt these gluteus muscle fixing and reinforcing activities to treat back uneasiness.

- You'll be practically off the chair if you lift just one glute.
- Perform a 30-second rocking motion from side to side.
- Next, work your gluteus muscles.
- Ten seconds must be spent in that position.
- You cat tone your glute, making arabesque circles while on the phone. They were initially intended for dancers only! If you have your own office, you can do this best.
- Your feet should be shoulder-width apart.
- Lift your left leg in front of you, shifting your weight to the right leg
- Slowly circle your left leg 10 times clockwise and 10 times in the counterclockwise directions.
- Alter your legs.

8. Workouts with a water bottle

A dumbbell can be substituted for a full water bottle. Take a sip if someone interrupts you.
- Sit up straight and contract your abs.
- With your right hand, twist the water bottle upward toward your shoulder.
- Repeat fifteen more times.
- Change arms.
- You can also perform overhead presses, and front arm lifts with your water bottle.
- Bend your elbows with the bottle in your right hand
- Raise your arm to the sky.
- Rep from the opposing side.
- Water bottle turns are a great method to thin down.

9. Exercises that can be done at a conference table to tone and strengthen your muscles.

To do toning and strengthening exercises at a conference table:
- Start by raising the table
- Place your hand under the table and push your body into it
- Use one hand, and repeat until your muscles are sore
- Place your palms down on the table and apply as much pressure as you can, then stop when your muscles are tired. The goal is to push the table into the ground.

If you want it to look more natural, you can do this with just one hand or two.
- In this exercise, you can practice answering "I don't know" with a shoulder shrug.
- Bring your shoulders up close to your ears.
- Keep it there for three to five seconds.
- Relax.

This move will make you appear focused while also working your entire body.
- To do an exercise that works your legs and upper body:
- Sit on the edge of a chair
- Place both hands on the table, press down, and lift your legs up as high as possible.

10. Static strength training:

To do some isometric exercises that can be done discreetly at your computer:
- Make a fist and squeeze it

- Hold before letting go
- Spread your fingers out
- Repeat ten times. Using a stress ball is optional. These exercises can help relax your fingertips if you spend a lot of time typing.

To strengthen your calves while reading or listening to a podcast:
- Stand in front of the chair and cling to it
- Place your right foot against the back of your left calf
- Lift your toes off the ground and hold the position for 20-30 seconds
- Repeat 5 times for each leg.

Kegel exercises are a way to strengthen the muscles in the pelvic floor to prevent or control incontinence. They can be done discreetly while you are doing your normal work. To do Kegel exercises:
- Contract your pelvic floor muscles
- Hold for five seconds
- Relax
- Repeat three times a week, five times a day.

This squeeze-hold-release technique can be used to strengthen almost any muscle.

11. Non-exercising Calorie Takers

Sometimes, the simplest way to burn calories is not to exercise at all. Here are a few non-exercise weight loss strategies.
- When at all possible, stand. For a person who weighs 155 pounds, you'll burn up to 50 extra calories per hour by moving around instead of sitting.

- You can burn an additional 350 calories each day by fidgeting. It counts to quickly tape your foot, talk with your hands, and chew gum. Even though each movement only burns a few calories, fidgeting can help you lose up to 36 pounds (or 16.3 kilograms) in a year.
- A great way to strengthen your core is to adopt a good posture. You need to use your muscles to keep your back straight and your belly taut. Perform it on a regular basis to improve your confidence, strengthen your abdominal muscles, and alleviate lower back pain.

When you breathe deeply, you will feel more relaxed due to the slowing of blood pressure.

Solve Your Health Problems with These Simple Exercises

Depression

Physical activity isn't a panacea for depression; None exists. However, numerous studies have demonstrated that physical activity can lessen or even eliminate depressive symptoms.

Those who suffer from depression and other health conditions appear to benefit significantly from exercise for their mental health and the quality of their life when used in conjunction with standard treatment. According to the researchers, the more exercise you do, the better.

Certain brain chemicals that aid in the formation of new brain cells and new connections between brain cells can be enhanced by exercise.

Exercise has several benefits for physical health and mental health. It can improve cardiovascular fitness, metabolic health, and brain health, and it can help boost self-esteem and self-efficacy by allowing you to set and achieve small goals, such as walking for half an hour.

Exercise is an important component of overall well-being and can effectively improve both physical and mental health. Exercising in a group or with a friend or partner can also improve your social connections.

Whether you need assistance increasing your level of physical activity or simply want to try out new hobbies, the following workouts may help alleviate symptoms of depression.

Run for a mood boost that is all-natural.

Exercise has been shown to affect certain brain chemicals and can lead to a feeling of euphoria, often referred to as a "runner's high, caused by the endorphins produced in the brain thanks to that exercise. Many athletes report experiencing a runner's high after reaching a certain level of exertion.

Endorphins make the body feel good and reduce pain perception. Exercise has many physical benefits, including lessening muscle tension, improving sleep quality, and lessening anxiety. To overcome depression, you can swim, run, walk, dance, or ski. You can reduce depressive symptoms by 25-30 minutes a day. Even a 10 to 15 minute burst of activity can help if you're short on time.

Anxiety

Often when you are stressed, you also start to become anxious. When anxiety becomes excessive, you begin to experience daily life poorly. If you're feeling anxious, try this exercise anytime and any place to find comfort. The idea is to do activities that will help you relax rapidly.

The exercise targets your body's stress responses, such as elevated heart rate, rapid breathing, and stiff muscles, and assists in replacing these with how your body feels when it is calm.

Breathe deeply to unwind.

Your heart rate and respiration rate may increase when you are anxious. You could likewise begin perspiring and feel mixed up or woozy. Controlling your breathing can help you relax your body and mind when you're stressed.

When you're anxious, take these steps to calm your breathing:

- Find a spot where you can relax and unwind. Put one hand on your chest and one on your stomach. When you take a big breath, your stomach should move more than your chest.
- Through your nose, slowly and steadily inhale. Pay attention to and feel your hands as you inhale. Your stomach hand should move slightly while your chest hand should remain motionless.
- Gradually breathe out through your mouth.
- It would be best if you did this at least ten times until you notice a reduction in your anxiety.

Abdominal Fat

It is difficult to get rid of the stubborn fat in your abdomen. To lose belly fat, you must perform specific activities. People with belly fat are more likely to get heart disease, diabetes, stroke, and some malignancies. Combat abdominal fat by exercising and making lifestyle changes.

Crunches

Crunches are the most efficient exercise for burning tummy fat. When it comes to fat-burning workouts, crunches come in the first place. This exercise will likewise support the improvement of abs while diminishing stomach fat.

What to Do
- Rests on a mat with your knees flexed and your feet on the floor.
- Place one thumb behind each ear. With the remaining fingers, grasp the back of your head. Raise your head off the floor. This is your starting point.
- Begin by curling up and attempting to reach your knees with your head.
- Return to your starting point.
- Inhale while curling up and exhale while curling down. Perform two sets of 12 repetitions.

What Not To Do
- Avoid tucking your chin in.

Stroke

Stroke exercises are important for stroke survivors looking to restore their mobility. According to research, there is a critical time period following a stroke of up to 6-8 months when the most recovery happens with rehabilitation. However, there is evidence that neuroplasticity persists throughout life. In fact, a continuous home exercise regimen is one of the most effective strategies to prolong therapy after leaving inpatient rehabilitation.

Strength, stride, and balance can all be improved through leg stroke exercises for survivors. The risk of falling, which is something that all stroke survivors want to avoid, can also be reduced through leg training.

Extensions of the Knee

Begin in a seated position with appropriate postural alignment for this leg workout. Then, straighten your leg by extending it while squeezing your thigh (quadriceps) muscles. Hold for 3 seconds, then carefully lower your foot to the floor. Repeat with your left leg (10 repetitions on each leg). Maintain your posture during the activity.

Migraines and tension headaches

If you suffer from migraine headaches daily, you may be seeking strategies to alleviate them. After all, having a migraine might make it difficult to perform regular tasks. These stretches can help relieve migraine symptoms by relieving tension in your upper body. They're also simple and soft, making them excellent for migraine sufferers.

Stretching on a regular basis can assist in soothing the body and mind. Yoga is a workout that incorporates stretching, breathing, and awareness. This may alleviate stress and tension, two major migraine triggers. Stretching helps to relax your muscles and relieve physical tension. This can also help with migraine attacks, as physical tension can exacerbate pain and stress.

The neck bends to the side

You can reduce tension in your upper back and neck by doing lateral neck bending exercises. It's a versatile maneuver because you can do it while sitting or standing.

To perform the stretch:

- Begin in either a seated or standing position. Maintain a neutral spine, relax your shoulders, and place your arms beside your body.
- Lower your right ear toward your right shoulder. Extend your left hand toward the floor and bend your fingers upward. Hold the position for 30 seconds.
- Return to the starting point. Repeat on the opposite side.

Chronic shoulder and neck pain

Neck and shoulder pain, like other types of chronic pain, can be addressed with a combination of natural therapies and good behaviors. Hot and cold therapy, stretching and strengthening exercises, and good posture are all highly recommended.

Stretching and strengthening can reduce pain while also strengthening muscles to prevent future injuries. If you experience any additional pain while performing these simple exercises, stop immediately and consult a healthcare expert.

Neck pain relief stretches

Here are three easy stretches for neck pain.
- Keep your shoulders straight and lower your chin to your chest. For 15 to 30 seconds, hold the stretch. Relax and slowly return your chin to its starting position.
- Maintain straight shoulders and tilt your head to one side. Stand still for 30 seconds. Relax and slowly get back into the starting position. On the opposing side, respond.
- Make sure your ear is facing your shoulder by tilting your head. Stand still for about 30 seconds. Slowly revert to your original posture after you relax. Turn your head to the other side to do it again.

Use these stretches to warm up before doing your strengthening exercises.

Neck pain cure strengthening exercises

Here are two exercises that will help you avoid future neck pain and injuries:

- Hold your shoulder blades together for 5 seconds. Squeeze gently; it should feel comfortable. Repeat 10 times every day.
- Lean back to dumb, open your feet to shoulder width, and perform a push-up, trying to keep your neck straight. Perform 10 reps twice a day with 2 sets.

Shoulder pain stretching exercises

These stretches help to release the tight muscles that cause discomfort and also improve flexibility to help prevent future injuries.

- Tuck your chin slightly forward, then slowly pull it back toward your throat. Maintain a parallel chin to the floor. Do this up to ten times each hour.
- Maintain an erect posture with a modest bend in your upper back. Now, roll your shoulders up, back, and down in a flowing circle. Do this for 10 repetitions, then swap directions and roll your shoulders forward for 10 repetitions.

Use these stretches to warm up before doing your strengthening exercises.

Shoulder pain strengthening exercises

These two examples of strengthening exercises use little to no equipment to help prevent shoulder soreness.

- Fill a water bottle (1.5 liters or so) to around 30 percent capacity.

- Raise your arm and hold it at shoulder height for about 1 minute.
- Switch arms three times on each side.
- Lie on your stomach, arms at your sides. If necessary, place a pillow beneath your brow.
- Bring your shoulder blades together and toward your feet gently.
- Hold for 10 seconds after relaxing your shoulders halfway down.
- Return to the starting position and perform the exercise 10 times.
- Working on your posture might also help you avoid neck and shoulder problems.

Asthma

Many people, except for those with severe asthma, take breathing for granted. Your lungs' airways become narrowed because of asthma, making it difficult to breathe. Corticosteroids and beta-agonists taken by mouth open your airways, easing breathing. However, these medications may not be enough to control symptoms for some people with severe asthma.

If you wish to augment your pharmacological treatment, you might want to attempt breathing exercises. Until recently, doctors would not offer breathing exercises for asthma patients since there was insufficient evidence that they worked. However, current research suggests that these workouts may assist in improving your breathing and quality of life. Based on current data, breathing exercises may be helpful as an adjunct therapy to medication and other basic asthma treatments.

Breathing through the diaphragm

Under your lungs is a muscle called the diaphragm that helps you breathe. It has a dome shape. Learning to breathe from your diaphragm rather than your chest is known as diaphragmatic breathing. Your diaphragm will be strengthened, your breathing will slow down, and your body will need less oxygen from this method.

To practice breathing through the diaphragm:
- Sit up straight in a chair.
- Your stomach and upper chest should be flattened by one hand.
- Breathe deeply into your nose slowly. The hand on your chest should remain fixed, while the hand on your stomach should move.
- Exhale slowly with pursed lips.
- Continue to practice this method until you can breathe in and out without your chest moving.

Bronchitis

Bronchitis patients often have significant breathing problems, so they need exercises to strengthen the chest muscles and open the airways.

Some workouts that may be beneficial for patients with chronic bronchitis (a subset of chronic obstructive lung disease) include:

- **Yoga.**
  Yoga's signature breath work and mild stretching can be an excellent way to improve your entire body, but especially your chest muscles and other portions of your respiratory tract.

- **Swimming.**

Swimming and water aerobics is a great exercise against bronchitis because:
- the warm air helps you breathe easier
- it increases your lung capacity through cardiovascular training
- it allows you to exercise almost all the muscles in your body.

But try to choose a ventilated and clean swimming pool because Chloramine levels in excess can cause breathing problems in some people

- **Walking.**

A quick walk outside in the fresh air can also help to loosen up the airways and improve your capacity to breathe easily.

- **Cycling.**

Cycling, like swimming and walking, provides cardiovascular advantages while being mild on the joints. These lower-body exercises benefit those suffering from bronchitis or other lung disorders. They are the same as those used in physiotherapy courses.

For those suffering from severe chronic bronchitis, this physical therapy will focus on the lungs to help increase the patient's ability to breathe. It consists of breathing exercises, stretching, and light aerobic training aimed to improve lung capacity and relieve congested breathing.

Insomnia

Many people have trouble falling asleep, but it's usually much easier after a little exercise. It is true, but you need not swim for 30 minutes or run 5 miles to enjoy this benefit. You can consistently get a superior night's rest with just 10 minutes of moderate movement. The cycle of sleep and wakefulness can be normalized by exercising in the morning or later in the day. The exercise makes the body warmer, which makes it easier to fall and stay asleep. Five exercises that will help you sleep better are listed below.

Yoga and extending

Yoga may not seem like a very remarkable exercise; however, a thorough 30-minute yoga meeting might consume somewhere in the range of 150 and 200 calories. Your body's temperature rises with each movement, which helps you regulate your sleep cycle. Additionally, quiet breathing at the end of a yoga practice helps the body relax. Yoga poses like the plank, chair, and high lunge are great for making your heart rate faster and burning more calories. After a yoga class, try chest-to-knees, cobbler's position, spinal twist, or corpse pose to unwind. By clearing your mind, this workout will help you sleep better.

Walking

Even though it may seem obvious, many people fail to recognize its significance. Strolling should be possible in a recreation area or on your own patio. A gym's treadmill is another great place to walk. How quickly you want to walk is up to you. You can walk leisurely around the block or vigorously through the park. You can swing your arms with some small hand weights, which is a bonus. A good walk, especially one that is taken outside, is not only good for your health but also helps you relax. You can enjoy the clean air and feel the warm breeze on your face. Endorphins, powerful brain chemicals that aid in sleep, are released during a pleasant walk.

Menopause and Hot Flashes

Every woman goes through menopause in her own unique way. Some people experience modest symptoms that resolve rapidly. Others have an outburst of hot flashes and mood changes. The good news is that you can make lifestyle modifications to help you manage the changes in your body. In addition to reducing menopausal symptoms, regular exercise is also an excellent strategy to avoid weight gain and muscle loss, which are two common menopausal complaints.

Cardio

It's good to do aerobic exercise that keeps your heart rate steady while working your big muscles. Your cardio options are almost limitless. You can walk, swim, run, or take a bike ride!

I recommend you start with 15 minutes daily and increase the time as you get more trained.

Meditation and yoga

To get relief from menopause, you can use yoga or meditation. These relaxation techniques can be customized for each woman, such as deep breathing, yoga, or meditation. Yoga positions that are supported and restorative may provide some assistance. These poses might help you relax by concentrating your mind. They can also assist with symptoms like:

- flashes of heat
- irritability
- fatigue

Exercises for Your Vagus Nerve

Massage Therapy for Your Vagus Nerve

The vagus nerve functions as a communication highway, monitoring your health state via various signals. There are numerous advantages to activating your vagus nerve, including headache and migraine relief, stress and anxiety reduction, improved digestion, and inflammation reduction. To reactivate it, gently massage your neck, shoulders, feet, or stomach.

Here are how and where to massage your body to stimulate your vagus nerve and understand the massage spots

1. Massage of the stomach vagus nerve

To be practiced on an empty stomach, this abdominal massage technique is simple to perform at home in a matter of minutes. However, you should begin cautiously and observe how your body reacts to the massage:

- Lie down on a soft floor mat or bed.
- Put your hands beneath your breastbone. Make soft downward stroking motions with your hands, bringing them down toward your abdomen for a few minutes.

- Make little circular strokes with your fingertips on your abdomen. Proceed gradually deeper, applying intense yet comfortable pressure and working inward and downward. Continue for a few minutes.

2. Massage of the vagus nerve in the ear

Here are the three parts of the ear you can massage to stimulate the vagus nerve

- To relieve headaches and migraines, massage the top of the ear (the part attached to the head.
- To relieve migraine, you can also massage the cartilaginous part above the opening of the ear canal. Piercing this area can also stimulate the vagus nerve.
- To relieve earache and headache, gently massage the upper part of the lobe.

3. Neck massage for the vagus nerve

It is the simplest type of massage because you can rub practically anywhere to activate your vagus nerve. All you need is 10 minutes!

Massage your muscles under the head and up to the trapezius and sternocleidomastoid muscles; you can help yourself with slight twists.

Also, if you press with your fingers on the sides of your neck, you can give an excellent carotid sinus massage.

4. Massage of the feet to stimulate the vagus nerve

Many vagus nerve reflexes (or acupressure spots) are mapped on the feet. You can give yourself a foot massage by turning your ankle, stroking your sole in small strokes, and softly moving your toes back and forth.

Stretching Exercise for Your Vagus Nerve

There are a few different ways to stimulate the vagus nerve that can be enjoyable, calming, or part of your daily routine. There are a lot of choices for you. You do not have to complete each one; instead, select activities that excite you and make you happy.

1. Using a neck stretch to tone the vagus muscle can cause happy feelings because it sends the brain messages of safety. A simple neck massage stretches the sternocleidomastoid, a large muscle that runs along the side of your neck. Many of us are always tight. Simply rest your right hand on top of your head and gradually incline your head and right ear toward your right shoulder. Hold your gaze up for thirty seconds before moving on to the opposite side.

2. Stretching the torso activates the vagus nerve.

The torso exercise stimulates the vagus nerve by moving the rib cage and calming the nervous system. Sit on the floor or in a chair and twist around. Put your right hand outwardly of your abandoned leg and your left hand. Over your left shoulder, look. Lengthen your spine on the inhale; intensify the twist on the exhale. Then reverse sides.

3. To let go of the body and mind, you need to exhale.

Your vagus nerve will be stimulated by simply exhaling for a longer period. In fact, several studies found that deep, slow breathing for two minutes increased vagus nerve activity, resulting in a longer interval between heartbeats. This could improve one's capacity for making decisions! As indicated carefully, expanding the breathed-out breath conveys a correspondence to the mind through the vagus nerve that your body might settle down, prompting both physical and mental calm, and may try and incite rest.

4. Gargling with water for 30 seconds to 1 minute twice a day can help stimulate the vagus nerve.

5. Singing along to your favorite songs can also be beneficial, even if you don't have a great singing voice.

6. Laughing out loud, watching a funny movie or TV show, or spending time with someone who makes you laugh, can help stimulate the parasympathetic nervous system.

7. Writing down three things you are grateful for before bed or when you wake up can be a helpful way to stimulate the PNS.

8. Spending time enjoying beautiful things like watching a sunset, being in nature, looking at beautiful pictures, or playing with pets. These activities can help promote relaxation and improve overall well-being. It has been demonstrated that anything that elicits positive emotions, which varies from person to person, increases vagal tone and contributes to excellent physical health.

Yoga Exercise for the Vagus Nerve

The significance of the vagus nerve has garnered more attention in recent years. It is an essential component of the parasympathetic system (also called the "relax and digest" system). Heart rate and digestion also depend on it.

Our vagus nerve's "tone" is important to our overall health and well-being. Vagal tone is a natural instrument that addresses the action of the vagus nerve. The parasympathetic nervous system is activated when vagal tone or vagus nerve activity is increased, allowing us to relax after stressful situations. The activity of our vagal tone is strongly linked to feeling happy, so a higher vagal tone indicates a healthier mind and body. Increasing vagal tone can be accomplished in various practical ways through yoga, deep belly breathing, cold exposure, exercise, and meditation.

1. Deep Diaphragmatic Breath Meditation: Sit comfortably somewhere quiet and unbothered to begin. Relax your shoulders and put one hand on your lap and one on your stomach. Feel your abdomen press into your hand as you inhale to start practicing deep diaphragmatic breathing. While concentrating on the sensation of the breath, continue to breathe from the abdomen. Here, meditate for five to ten minutes. At the point when your psyche meanders, delicately and non-judgmentally take it back to the breath however many times as required. Then re-open your eyes.

2. The posture of a Youngster: Sit out of sorts, spread your knees wide, and bring your hands to the floor, taking deep breaths. While remaining in the child's pose, take a deep diaphragmatic breath in this shape for ten counts.

3. Forward Folding: Stand upright and spread your feet shoulder-width apart. Bend your torso until your hands rest on the floor (if you can)! As you relax into the pose and rest your tummy on

your thighs, allow your arms to hang heavily and encourage a slight knee bend. Relax your neck and bring your head down toward the mat. Ten times, take a deep breath.

4. Heart Opener Supported: Place a bolster or rolled blanket vertically in the middle of your mat if you don't already have one. While lying on your back, place the short edge of the support at your tailbone to open up your heart area. You can either spread your legs wide or bring your feet together for a reclining butterfly stance. Hold for ten counts, then take a deep breath.

5. Waterfall: Remove the support and place a block on your mat under your tailbone. Enter the waterfall pose by extending your legs toward the ceiling while keeping your knees slightly bent. While the rest of your body sinks into the dirt, let your legs be soft and relaxed. Stretch your ankles by twirling your feet. Ten deep inhalations

6. Happy baby: Lie on your mat and remove the block. Extend your legs toward the ceiling and grip the outside edges of your feet to get your knees closer to your armpits. Breathe deeply into your inner hips as you firmly root down into your spine. Hold the position for about 15 seconds to stretch the hamstrings. Ten deep inhalations

7. Savasana: Lie on your back in a supine position while extending your arms and legs far and wide. Breathe deeply in through your nose and out through your mouth a few times. By letting go of any attempts to control your breathing or thoughts, your body can release any tension it may be carrying. After taking in the results of your practice, you can stay here for up to ten minutes before gently leaving and returning to your day.

8. Relax Your Neck to Improve Vagus Nerve Health: The vagus nerve runs just below the sternocleidomastoid (SCM) muscles and in front of the scalenes, which are the tightest muscles in

the neck. Gentle stretching of the SCM and scalenes in the neck also produces a relaxing response via vagus nerve activation.

- Experiment with bringing your right ear to your right shoulder without twisting your head. Then, turn your gaze to the right.
- Take 4 or 5 deep breaths into the left side of your neck, then return your head to the center as your eyes return to the front.
- Repeat on the left side and take note of how you feel.
- You might also try bringing your right ear to your right shoulder while sending your eyes and looking to the left. Hold this shape for another 4 or 5 breaths before switching sides.

Vagus Nerve Acupressure Points

What Are Acupressure And Acupuncture?

Acupressure and acupuncture entail applying pressure to particular places on the body to stimulate your vagus nerve.

A licensed expert inserts special needles into the exact points of stimulation through acupuncture.

In contrast, acupressure can be practiced independently with the fingers or thumb.

It's also free to do.

Acupressure and acupuncture are efficient techniques for activating the vagus nerve, which has been found to enhance both physical and mental health in various ways. Below are three vagus nerve acupressure spots that you may execute fast and easily at home, along with a comprehensive list of advantages.

Acupressure & Acupuncture Benefits

Acupressure and acupuncture stimulate the vagus nerve, which Through the stimulations of the vagus nerve and the activation of the parasympathetic rest and digest system, you will be able to:

- relax your body
- increase your attention and memory during the day
- improve sleep during the night
- reduce frequent pain and inflammation
- reduce reed and tension by lowering your heart rate

Vagus Nerve Pressure Points

The vagus nerve can be stimulated through pressure at particular points to improve digestion and relieve the feeling of nausea and vomiting:

- The concha cymba at the ear
- Nei Guan P6 at the wrist/forearm
- Shin-Stomach 36

Press downward with your thumb, and then make circular movements for a couple of minutes. If you need to yawn or swallow, you have optimally activated the parasympathetic nervous system! Developing and maintaining new habits and routines can be challenging. However, acupressure may be practiced quickly and effortlessly at home while doing other things like watching TV or waiting for the kettle to boil, making it simple to add to your daily routine.

1. Ear - Concha Cymba

- Insert the finger into the ear
- Move your finger in a circular motion, exerting a slight pressure
- Repeat a couple of minutes for each ear

2. Wrist - Nei Guan P6

- Turn your hand over with the palm facing upward.

- Look for the two large tendons located below the wrist crease
- With the thumb of your other hand, apply a little pressure for a couple of minutes

3. Shin - Stomach 36

- Calculate 6 in/15 cm below your kneecap.
- Stomach 36 is located in the depression on this part above the shin.
- Press down on this spot and move your foot up and down.
- Make circular movements with your toe
- Repeat 2 minutes for each leg

Healthy and Unhealthy Food for Vagus Nerve and Beneficial Natural Supplements

Can the vagus nerve's activity be affected by what you eat and drink? The vagus nerve, which means "the wandering nerve" in Latin, connects the brain to the heart, lungs, and gastrointestinal tract, among other essential body systems and organs. We do not have a lot of scientific data on how diet affects the vagal tone or how well the vagus nerve communicates with organs and systems. Rather than natural treatments like a vagus nerve diet, most current research on vagus nerve therapeutic intervention focuses on electrical vagal stimulation.

However, we know that generally healthy dietary choices improve vagal tone and support a healthy vagus nerve. Because the vagus nerve can detect inflammation and microbial metabolites (like butyrate) in the gut, we can also conclude that diets promoting good gut health may improve vagal tone.

Diet and Beneficial Nutrients for Vagus Nerve Health

A review of the literature on the impact of nutrition on heart rate variability (HRV), an indirect measure of vagal tone, revealed the following associations with higher vagal tone:

Omega-3 fatty acids, the Mediterranean diet, yogurt with added nutrients, pistachios, probiotic foods and supplements, red wine with polyphenols, but not spirits or beer, vitamin B12, foods high in choline, magnesium, calcium, sodium (salt), and choline-rich foods.

Although this list is not comprehensive, it provides some insight into the foods that may be beneficial for activating the vagus nerve. Fortunately, many of these foods and nutrients are already taken on a regular anti-inflammatory diet. As a result, you don't need to go out of your way to include foods that are good for the vagus nerve if you already eat a varied, nutrient-dense, and colorful diet.

The vagus nerve is aided by acetylcholine, which is the principal parasympathetic nervous system neurotransmitter. Choline, a precursor to acetylcholine, is available in various foods, and eating more of them may enhance vagal tone. Choline, which is needed to generate acetylcholine, the most abundant neurotransmitter in the body, is arguably the most important actor in vagus nerve health on this list. Choline is very necessary for numerous vagus nerve processes. You can easily find choline in foods such as red meat or poultry, liver, eggs, and fish. It is not strictly a vitamin but is still part of the B vitamins. Animal foods are the best sources of dietary choline; most plant alternatives have extremely low levels and may be poorly absorbed.

Fortunately, a high-quality phosphatidylcholine supplement may also provide choline (the name says it all) when the body requires it. When we take BodyBio PC, our bodies can choose whether to break it down into choline and phospholipids or use it whole in our cell membranes. Isn't it convenient?

Foods high in choline include Eggs, Seeds of sunflowers, Meat from organs, Red potatoes, kidney beans, Quinoa, fish, beef, chicken, and fish filets.

Consumption of Sodium and Vagal Tone

Salt is another crucial nutrient to mention. Heart rate variability (HRV) indicated that women on "heavy sodium" diets had higher vagal tone. This finding is consistent with recent studies showing that salt, specifically real, mineralized salt, is necessary for long-term health and wellness.

A nonrandomized clinical trial found that decreased sodium admission was related to bringing down the vagal volume, while high sodium consumption further developed HRV/vagal tone. Vagal tone was higher in those who were salt-sensitive (as evidenced by elevated blood pressure following sodium intake) than in those who were not. This does not mean you should consume a lot more salt, but it might be worthwhile to see if your current intake is excessive. Despite its long history of demonization in Western medicine, sodium is an essential electrolyte for nerve impulses, muscle contraction, and body water balance. One should not take too much, but not too little, either!

Foods to Avoid for a Healthy Vagal Tone

Although there isn't a lot of scientific research on the foods that affect the vagus nerve, a literature review found that trans-fat consumption was linked to lower HRV/vagal tone. Many issues, including obesity, weight gain, poor cardiovascular health, metabolic dysfunction, and others, have been linked to trans-fat consumption. Trans fat can be found in things you know are hurtful for you, like handled food sources, high-fat food varieties, cheap food, seared food varieties, handled heated merchandise, non-dairy espresso half and half, microwave popcorn, etc.

We are aware that the vagus nerve influences gut function. The vagus nerve controls digestion, gastrointestinal motility, and the release of digestive enzymes by connecting the brain to the gut. On the other hand, neurotransmitters are made in the intestines and sent to the brain via the vagus nerve to show changes in pain, memory, and mood, among other things. The vagus nerve can also detect inflammation and nutritional levels in the intestines.

We don't know for sure if bad gut health leads to less vagal activity or if less vagal activity leads to bad gut health. Both of these things may be true: Poor gut health (inflammation brought on by bad food, infection, etc.) for some people leads to a vagus nerve that doesn't work as well, which could cause mood or motility problems. Because persistent stress disrupts the parasympathetic neural system and the vagus nerve, some people may experience stomach issues. We could deduce that diets and foods that support gut health may also support vagus nerve health, given the strong connection between the two.

The following are examples of various gut health diets:

- The Paleo diet
  A low-fat, low-glycemic, and low-carbohydrate diet and the elementary diet are all forms of the Paleo diet. The Paleo diet is frequently recommended as the initial course of action for restoring gut health because it is the least restrictive and still eliminates many common foods that cause allergies and inflammation. Paleo may be a great place to start if you're looking for a diet targeting the vagus nerve.

- Produce that is high in antioxidants, minerals, and polyphenols (such as blueberries, leafy greens, cruciferous vegetables, and vibrant root vegetables), healthy fats like avocado and olive oil, refreshments (for example, espresso and green tea). These are instances of stomach well-disposed feasts that may likewise increment vagal tone. Numerous of the aforementioned "choline foods" also benefit gut health. Probiotic supplements can also help intestinal health (and a healthy vagal tone).

Food Recipes

Breakfast, Appetizers, and Snacks

1. Breakfast Bowls with Cottage Cheese

These breakfast bowls with cottage cheese are a quick and healthy option for breakfast! Berries or apples, Cinnamon, and honey, drizzled on top.

Ingredients

- 1/2 to 3/4 cup chopped fresh berries or apples
- 3/4 cup cottage cheese
- 1 teaspoon cinnamon
- 2 tablespoons chopped pistachios or pecans
- 1 tablespoon honey

Instruction

1. Top with honey, berries, almonds, and cinnamon.
2. Consume right away.

2. Recipe for Challah French toast

This recipe for Challah French toast elevates breakfast to a whole new level. The bread has the best texture and flavor of custard.

Ingredients

- 1 1/2 cups milk
- 2 teaspoons sugar
- 2 teaspoons 1 teaspoon ground cinnamon
- 1 teaspoon ground nutmeg
- 1/8 teaspoon kosher salt
- 8 slices of one-inch-thick challah bread
- 1 tablespoon vanilla extract butter for cooking

Instructions

1. Whisk together the eggs, milk, sugar, vanilla, cinnamon, nutmeg, and kosher salt in a large bowl.
2. In a small pan, melt 1 tablespoon of butter over medium heat. 4 pieces of bread should be soaked in the egg mixture for about 15 seconds on each side or until they are saturated.
3. Brown the bread for two to three minutes on each side in the heated skillet.
4. Continue with the remaining bread slices and butter. Maple syrup and powdered sugar can be added right away, or you can toss both sides in cinnamon sugar according to Cinnamon French Toast's instructions.
5. Use whole milk for the most flavor. For a delicious twist, mix heavy cream with half the milk.

3. Oatmeal Baked with Pumpkin

This oatmeal baked with pumpkin is ideal for breakfast in the fall: packed with healthy oats and a spicy kick! Bake a pan and consume it for a week.

Ingredients:

- 2 cups old-fashioned rolled oats
- 1 1/2 cups chopped or whole pecans
- 1 teaspoon baking powder
- 12 teaspoons kosher salt
- 1 cup pureed pumpkin
- 14 cups chosen milk
- 6 tablespoons pure maple syrup
- 1 tablespoon melted and room temperature coconut oil
- 1 tablespoon pure vanilla extract
- 1 tablespoon melted coconut oil
- 1 tablespoon maple Greek yogurt

Instructions

4. Combine the rolled oats, pecan bits, baking powder, pumpkin spice, and kosher salt in a bowl.
5. Place the dried goods in the pan that has been prepared.
6. Combine the milk, maple syrup, coconut oil, vanilla extract, and pumpkin puree in the same mixing bowl. Pour that mixture over the oats and stir to ensure that everything is thoroughly incorporated.
7. Bake for 40 to 45 minutes the cake from the oven and cool it for 10 minutes.
8. Top with maple Greek yogurt and a drizzle of maple syrup before serving.
9. In a mixing bowl, combine 12 cups of Greek yogurt, 1 tablespoon of maple syrup, and 12 teaspoons of vanilla essence.

Apply a thin coating of maple syrup to the top before serving.
10. Apply a thin coating of maple syrup to the top before serving.

---

4. French Toast Sticks

This French toast sticks dish is enjoyable and simple to prepare at home! For a delightful special breakfast, roll them in cinnamon sugar. Looking for a creative breakfast idea? This French Toast Sticks recipe is exactly what you're looking for!

Ingredients

- 6 slices of Texas toast (or day-old bread)
- ¼ cup milk
- 2 eggs
- 1 teaspoon of sugar
- 1 teaspoon of vanilla extract
- ⅛ teaspoons of salt
- two tablespoons of butter are all needed to make the French toast.
- To make the Cinnamon sugar, one cup of granulated sugar and 1 teaspoon of ground cinnamon are needed

Instructions:

1. If possible, cover the bread with a napkin and let it sit at room temperature overnight. Because of this, the bread can maintain its dippable stick shape while maintaining a firmer texture.
2. Cut each slice of bread into four long sticks (leave the crust on).

3. Mix the eggs, sugar, vanilla, cinnamon, milk, and salt in a medium bowl. Mix the cinnamon sugar together and distribute it evenly on a plate to prepare it.
4. In a large skillet or griddle, melt the butter.
5. Work one stick at a time by quickly dipping it in the egg mixture until it covers all sides and shaking it off. In the heated skillet, arrange each in a batch the size of your frying surface.
6. Cook for a few minutes on each side, depending on the heat of the skillet and how many sticks you are cooking at once.
7. Roll the sticks in the cinnamon sugar as soon as they are finished. Serve immediately with syrup for dipping.

Notes:

- Avoid using spongy sandwich bread that you just bought because it won't stand up to the egg mixture and frying. When making the bread, keep the following considerations in mind:
- Using bread from the day before is beneficial. Leaving the bread out the prior night brings about a harder, more grounded surface, particularly for innately soft breads. With Texas toast, we tried both methods, but day old came out on top. Texas toast can be used the day before, but the bread is a little floppier.)
- Use Texas toast whenever possible. Because of its thick cut, this bread works well and forms attractive rectangle shapes.

- Alternately, use sourdough or another artisan bread with a firm texture. Because the texture can withstand and remain stiffer than that of other types of bread, this is also effective. The stick shapes will change due to the bread's shape. Indeed, putting the bread out for the time being makes a difference.)
- Keep the crusts on the sticks when chopping them. The sticks' structural stability is improved by the crusts.

---

5. Cranberry orange muffins

Combine with tart berries and zingy orange zest is these moist, sweet cranberry orange muffins. They are perfect!

Ingredients

- 2 cups of universal flour (280 grams)
- 2/3 cup sugar
- 1 teaspoon of ground cinnamon
- 1 tbsp of baking powder
- 1/2 teaspoon salt
- 2 eggs
- 1/4 cup of honey
- ½ cup of olive oil
- 1/2 cup of sour cream
- 1/2 cup of milk
- 1 tsp of apple cider vinegar
- 2 tbsp of orange zest (zest from 2 medium oranges)
- 1/2 cup of cranberries and additional ingredients for the topping.
- To make the glaze, 1 teaspoon of orange juice

Instructions

1. Spray cooking sprays a 12-cup muffin tin with muffin cups.
2. Get the batter ready: In the first bowl, combine the all-purpose flour, sugar, cinnamon, baking powder, and salt. In the second bowl, whisk the eggs with honey, yogurt, apple cider vinegar, orange zest, and vegetable oil until smooth. With a spatula, overlap the dry fixings into the wet parts until a thick, smooth player structure. The cranberries should be folded into the batter with a spatula.
3. Scoop the hitter equitably into the biscuit cups, filling them nearly to the top with a liberal ¼ cup for each biscuit. In a small bowl, combine a pinch of granulated sugar with a handful of the smallest cranberries, which should equal about 1/4 cup. Then drive them into the biscuit tops.
4. Bake for 20 to 22 minutes (on the preheated stove – 400°F)) or until the muffins are golden and puffy. After 5 minutes, transfer to a table for about 1 hour of cooling.
5. Make a thick icing by combining the powdered sugar and orange juice in a bowl before glazing. If the surface is excessively thick, add a couple of additional drops of squeezed orange and speed until it meets up; if it's excessively flimsy, add somewhat more sugar.

Using a fork, drizzle a small amount over each muffin.

6. If iced, store for approximately two days or four days at room temperature in a tightly sealed container. Unglazed can be stored in the refrigerator for up to a week at room temperature.

6. Pumpkin chocolate chip bread

This pumpkin chocolate chip bread is incredibly filling and delicious! Dark chocolate and warming spices work wonderfully together.

Ingredients

- 2 eggs
- 1 cup pureed pumpkin
- 2 cups unscented oil
- 1 tablespoon cinnamon
- 1 teaspoon vanilla extract
- 1 teaspoon ginger powder
- 1 teaspoon ground allspice
- 2 teaspoons ground cloves
- 3/4 teaspoon kosher salt
- 1 teaspoon baking powder baking soda
- half a cup of all-purpose flour (210 grams)
- one cup of semisweet or bittersweet chocolate chips (or mini, if desired).

Instructions

1. Spray cooking spray on a 9-inch aluminum bread pan.
2. In a bowl, whisk the eggs together. Then, at that point,

add the pumpkin puree, sugars, oil, and vanilla concentrate.

3. Mix the kosher salt, cinnamon, ginger, allspice, and cloves in a bowl. Then incorporate the baking soda and baking powder. Using a spatula, gradually add the flour, half at a time, until it is barely incorporated and there are no dry bits left (do not over-stir). Before gently folding the chips into the batter, toss one cup of them with one tablespoon of flour to prevent them from sinking.

4. Sprinkle the remaining 14 cups of chocolate chips on top of the batter, filling the bread pan to the halfway point.

5. Bake for about 1 hour, or until a toothpick inserted into the center comes out clean; 45 minutes before baking time, lightly cover the top with aluminum foil. The temperature inside ought to be in the range of 200°F and 205°F. In the pan, allow cooling to room temperature. After cutting around the edges with a knife, invert. Divide into serving pieces. The next day, the flavor and texture get better. It can be refrigerated for ten days (return to room temperature before serving) or frozen in slices for several months when wrapped in foil.

7. Fruit Dip in a Flash

Only three ingredients. It is easy to make and takes only 2 min to mix.

Ingredients:

- 1 cup plain Greek yogurt (whole milk)
- 1 tablespoon honey
- 1 teaspoon vanilla extract

Instructions:

Mix all the ingredients in a mixing dish. Serve immediately with fruit for dipping, or store for up to ten days in the refrigerator.

8. Delicious Sweet Potato Bites

The most delicious and popular healthy appetizer is these delicious potatoes!

Ingredients

- 1 cup of olive oil
- 1 teaspoon garlic powder
- 2 pounds of sweet potatoes
- 1 teaspoon chili powder
- 1 cup shredded cheddar cheese
- 1 teaspoon of chili powder, kosher salt, spicy sauce
- 3 green onions
- and sour cream

Instructions

1. Pre-heat the oven to 450°F
2. Slice sweet potatoes into 14-inch slices. To thoroughly coat both sides, place the slices in a bowl and toss with the olive oil,

chili powder, garlic powder, and kosher salt.

3. Line a baking sheet with parchment paper and place the rounds in an even layer. Bake for ten minutes on one side, then flip and bake for another ten minutes.

4. Meanwhile, slice the 3 onions.

5. Take the potatoes out of the oven and brush each round with hot sauce. Melt the cheese on top of every round for a few minutes.

6. Serve the rounds on a large dish. Sliced green onions and a dollop of sour cream should be added to each round. Tip: Mix a few drops of water into the sour cream in a bowl to make it easier to spoon out.

9. Recipe for Cheese Balls

This traditional cheese ball recipe has a lot of flavor! Everyone at the party will gather around this easy appetizer.

Ingredients

- 16 ounces of room-temperature cream cheese
- 2 blocks
- 1 cup cheddar cheese
- 2 green onions
- 1 teaspoon Worcestershire sauce
- ¼ tsp of hot sauce
- ½ tsp garlic powder
- ½ tsp smoked paprika
- ¼ tsp dried dill
- ¼ tsp fit salt
- ¾ cup slashed toasted walnuts saltines for serving

Instructions

1. Permit the cream cheddar to come to room temperature prior to utilizing (let it stand around 30 minutes unrefrigerated or see the tips above). Beat the cream cheese for 30 seconds, or until smooth, on medium speed in a mixer.

2. In a mixing bowl, combine the kosher salt, Worcestershire sauce, garlic powder, smoked paprika, dried dill, hot sauce, and shredded cheddar cheese. Thinly slice the onions. Reserve 1 tablespoon of the finely chopped greens and then mix on low speed until combined.

3. Place the cheese on a piece of plastic wrap with a spoon. Roll the cheese into a ball and cover it with plastic wrap. Set aside for one hour.

4. Toast the pecans in an oil-free, dry skillet over medium heat for about 4 minutes until the nuts are fragrant and slightly darker. Set aside on a tray after taking it out of the heat. Finely chop the pecans before placing them in a shallow bowl. Include the remaining chopped green onions.

5. Delicately roll the cheddar ball in the walnut blend, squeezing daintily to cover the whole ball. Before serving, allow 30 minutes at room temperature.

If needed, you can freeze for up to a month (wrapped tightly in foil and plastic wrap) or refrigerate for up to two weeks.

10. Cheese and charcuterie board

It consists of cheeses, marinated vegetables, cured meats, olives, and other Italian antipasti.

Ingredients

- Mozzarella Balls, marinated (or purchased)
- 1 cup seasoned mushrooms
- 1 cup mixed olives, blocks of aged cheese
- 1 cup roasted peppers, various types of cured meats (prosciutto, salami, chorizo, bresaola, etc.)
- 1 cup cherry tomatoes and 2 tablespoons. crackers 1 tablespoon Italian breadsticks Other optional components: roasted almonds, canned pepperoncini, and other similar items

Instructions

1. If making your own, make the marinated mozzarella balls and/or mushrooms.
2. If necessary, prepare the remaining ingredients: Place the cheddar or meats in little dishes, then the olives and nuts in bigger dishes.
3. The items should be placed on a large cutting board. First, fill the bowls with crackers, breadsticks, marinated vegetables, cheese slices, and meats. To finish the tray, add a few fresh herb sprigs, such as rosemary or thyme sprigs, once the board is mostly finished.
4. If desired, serve immediately with toothpicks, small plates, and forks. The antipasto dish can be left out for up to two hours at room temperature.

11. Mushroom Galette

This robust mushroom galette is a delicious and flavorful recipe for a savory tart. This vegetarian meal idea will impress everyone.

Ingredients

The mixture for the galette
- [210 grams] 1 ½cups broadly useful flour, evened out and spooned
- ¾ genuine salt teaspoon
- 1/4 teaspoon baking powder
- 10 tablespoons margarine
- 5 to 6 teaspoons of cold water
- Flaky Ocean salt for use as a topping

For the filling
- 16 ounces of cleaned and cut cremini mushrooms
- 4 ounces Shiitake mushrooms, cut and with the stems eliminated
- 2 tablespoons Olive oil
- a serving of soy sauce (or tamari)
- 2 tablespoons Garlic powder
- 1 teaspoon of powdered onion
- 1 teaspoon paprika

- 1/2 tsp. dried thyme
- 1/4 teaspoon kosher salt and more salt for garnish
- 3/4 cup whole milk ricotta
- shredded Parmesan cheese
- 1 tiny clove of grated garlic,
- freshly ground pepper
- 2 fresh thyme sprigs for garnish

Instructions

1. Cut the butter into the flour mixture until it is mostly mixed and has a texture like peas.
2. Mix the flour and four tablespoons of the cool water until most of the flour is incorporated. Add the additional 1 to 2 tablespoons of water and knead the dough with your fingers. Avoid adding additional water; It ought to be combined already. By rolling the dough into a ball and flattening it, you can make a thick disk. The batter ought to cool for an hour prior to being enclosed by plastic or set in a shut holder. (The dough can be made up to three days in advance; before rolling, let it sit for 30 minutes at room temperature.
3. The oven should be heated to 400 degrees.
4. It is necessary to clean and cut the mushrooms. Combine the soy sauce, smoked paprika, olive oil, garlic powder, onion powder, thyme, and 12 teaspoons of kosher salt in a bowl. Line a baking sheet, arrange them in a single layer, and bake for 15 min.
5. In a mixing bowl, combine the ricotta, Parmesan, garlic, 14 teaspoons of kosher salt, and a pinch of black pepper.
6. Lightly flour the table and stretch the dough on it into a 12-inch circle, leaving the edges unpolished (if necessary, move the dough around and add a little more flour underneath to prevent it from sticking). Line a rimmed baking sheet with a piece of parchment paper and transfer it to the dough.
7. Before adding the mushrooms and laying the ricotta mixture on top, leave at least 2 inches of dough around the outside border. Fold the dough's outside edges over the filling to form a crust about 2 inches thick, overlapping the folds as shown in the images. On top, add some more thyme leaves.
8. After whisking, apply the egg mixture to the crust with a pastry brush. The crust is then sprinkled lightly with flaky sea salt for the final touch.
9. After 30 to 33 minutes of baking, the crust should be golden brown. Place the parchment paper on a cooling rack after removing it from the oven. After at least ten minutes of cooling, slice into pieces and serve. It functions effectively, both warm and cold. Keep leftovers in the refrigerator up to three days; Reheat at room temperature or in the oven before serving.

12. Pumpkin French Toast

Make some pumpkin French toast with toasty spices and maple syrup sprinkled on top. It's light and delicious.

Ingredients:

- 4 eggs
- 1 1/2 cups milk
- 1 1/2 cups pumpkin puree
- 2 teaspoons sugar
- 1 teaspoon vanilla extract
- 1 teaspoon ground cinnamon
- 1 teaspoon Pumpkin pie spice
- 1/8 teaspoon kosher salt
- 10 slices of bread, cut to 3/4-inch thickness, from an Italian or French loaf, sourdough, challah, or brioche loaf
- 1 tablespoon Butter for cooking

Instructions:

1. In a large bowl, combine eggs, milk, pumpkin puree, sugar, vanilla, cinnamon, pumpkin spice, and kosher salt.
2. Soften 1 tablespoon spread on an iron over medium intensity. Four pieces of bread should be submerged in the egg mixture for 10 to 15 seconds on each side for artisan or sourdough bread.
3. Brown the bread for two to three minutes on each side in the heated skillet.
4. Continue with the remaining bread slices and butter.
5. Serve promptly with maple syrup and a powdered sugar sprinkling.

Main Dishes

13. Mediterranean Tuna Salad

This quick and delicious Mediterranean tuna salad can be made for lunch or dinner in no time at all!

Ingredients

- 1 red bell pepper, roughly diced
- 1 cup English cucumber, chopped (or standard cucumber, peeled)
- 2 cans, 5 ounces white meat tuna
- 3 tablespoons of drained capers
- 1 tablespoon of white wine vinegar
- 1 tablespoon of extra virgin olive oil
- 1 tablespoon of olive oil Dijon mustard
- ¼ tsp legitimate salt
- 2 tbsp. crumbles of feta cheese (optional)

Instructions

1. Prepare the English cucumber, shallot, and red pepper.
2. In a small bowl, drain the tuna and crush it well. Add the chopped vegetables, capers, olive oil, Dijon mustard, feta (if using), kosher salt, and white wine vinegar to the bowl. Season with additional salt if desired. Refrigerate for as long as 3 days.

14. Kale Barley Salad

This vibrant kale and quinoa salad is loaded with healthy ingredients and tastes great!

Ingredients

- 2 cups of cooked barley
- 1 bunch of Lacinato kale
- 15 ounces of chickpeas that have been washed and drained
- 14 cups finely chopped red shallot
- 1 red bell pepper
- carrots
- 14 cups extra virgin olive oil
- 13 cup apple cider vinegar
- 1 tbsp. Dijon mustard,
- 1 teaspoon curry powder
- 1 clove of garlic
- 12 teaspoons kosher salt, and black pepper, to taste

Instructions

1. Cook the barley. Spread the barley in a single layer on a baking sheet and freeze it for 2 to 3 minutes to bring it to room temperature.
2. Preparation for Kale: Slice the kale. The kale should be sprinkled with one pinch of kosher salt. Brush each kale leaf with oil until they are supple in all areas.
3. Get the remaining vegetables ready: Finely chop the shallot or onion. Pepper and carrots should be diced.

4. Combine the ingredients for the dressing: In a medium mixing bowl, combine the curry powder, grated garlic, Dijon mustard, olive oil, and apple cider vinegar.
5. Combine the ingredients for the salad: With the dressing, 1/2 teaspoons of kosher salt, and freshly ground pepper, combine the vegetables, quinoa, and chickpeas. Add more kosher salt to taste.

15. Quick Hummus

Bowls Hummus bowls are a great way to eat lunch or dinner quickly: cooking is not required! Add toppings made of crisp vegetables to each dollop.

Ingredients

- 1 cup of hummus
- 8 slices of English cucumber (or standard cucumber, peeled)
- 1 handful of sliced cherry tomatoes
- 1 tablespoon Kalamata olives
- 1 tablespoon feta cheese (to sprinkle) (optional or use vegan feta for vegan)
- 1 handful of chopped baby greens or lettuce
- 1 cup of boiled rice or pre-cooked rice (optional)
- Easy Couscous or Easy Orzo
- 1 pita sandwich, pita chips, or gluten-free crackers

Instructions

1. If using, add the greens and rice to the bowl (for a quick shortcut, use packaged precooked rice). Season the rice with salt and a touch of olive oil if utilizing.
2. Top with olives, feta cheese, hummus, cucumber, tomato, and red onion slices. The vegetables can be dressed or dipped in hummus and pita wedges.

16. Biscuits with egg

This recipe for egg biscuits is incredible for a sound lunch! For quick meals, bake eggs in muffin cups and store them in the refrigerator.

Ingredients

- 6 large eggs
- 1/2 teaspoon dried oregano
- 1/2 teaspoon kosher salt
- 1 cup Parmesan cheese, grated
- 1/4 cup chopped roasted red pepper (jar); additional ingredients for garnish
- freshly ground black pepper
- Spray or lubricate a 12-cup muffin pan.

Instructions

1. Place the spinach in a colander and run warm water over it for 1 moment to defrost it. If necessary, you can also use a microwave. The next step is to squeeze them to extract all the liquid.

2. In a large mixing bowl, mix the eggs. The cottage cheese, oregano, salt, garlic powder, shredded Parmesan, spinach, and roasted red pepper should all be thoroughly mixed in. Whenever wanted, season with new ground dark pepper.

3. Fill approximately three-quarters of each muffin cup with the egg mixture. If desired, garnish with additional roasted red pepper.

4. Bake for about 25 minutes. Run a butter knife down the sides of each muffin to loosen and pop it out after a few minutes of cooling (they will deflate, which is normal). Enjoy right away or let it sit for up to five days: They can be rewarmed, eaten cold, or at room temperature. They can also be frozen and thawed overnight in the refrigerator for up to three months.)

5. Note:

6. To adjust the blend-ins in this recipe, supplant the spinach with 1 to 1 ½ cup blend-ins, roasted peppers and onions or sautéed peppers, sautéed mushrooms, finely diced ham or bacon, caramelized onions, sautéed broccoli, and so on. You want the vegetables to be done when you sauté them, so they don't lose too much moisture when baked.

17. Wraps of Lasagna

Wraps of lasagna are a novel way to serve this traditional dish! Make a delicious and entertaining dinner by wrapping the contents in noodles.

Ingredients

- 1/2 lasagna noodles (10 ounces)
- 1 grated garlic clove
- 2/8 ounces of fire-roasted crushed tomatoes
- 2 tablespoons olive oil
- 2 teaspoons dried oregano
- 12 teaspoons kosher salt
- 10 ounces of frozen spinach
- 2 tablespoons chopped fresh basil
- 15 ounces for garnish
- ricotta cheese
- 1/2 cup Parmesan cheese
- 1/2 teaspoon lemon zest
- 1 egg
- and parsley for garnish

Instructions

1. Heat up the noodles: Bring a large pot of salty water to a boil. Following the package's instructions, cook the noodles until just al dente, stirring frequently. Apply olive oil to a baking sheet after the noodles have been drained. To prevent the noodles from sticking, turn them over on the sheet and coat them with olive oil.

2. Meanwhile, set up the pureed tomatoes: In a bowl, combine the fire-roasted tomatoes, garlic, olive oil, 3/4 teaspoon

kosher salt, and 1 teaspoon dried oregano. Combine thoroughly until the olive oil is completely incorporated.

3. Get the filling ready: Follow the package's instructions to thaw the spinach, then use your fingers to extract all the water (the spinach should feel dry and crumbly before you use it). In the second mixing bowl, mix the basil, ricotta, Parmesan, 12 cups mozzarella, lemon zest, egg, 1 teaspoon dried oregano, 34 teaspoons kosher salt, and freshly ground pepper.

4. In a 9 x 13-inch pan, spread half of the tomato sauce on the bottom. Roll the noodles and set four noodles on a baking sheet. Cover with one cup of the cheese mixture. Place each noodle in the pan after gently rolling it. Continue with the other noodles.

5. Complete the pan: cover the noodles with the remaining 12 cups of mozzarella after they have been wrapped in the remaining tomato sauce.

6. Bake for twenty minutes with foil covering the pan but not touching the cheese. When the foil is removed, bake for ten minutes. If desired, broil the cheese for 2 minutes until it is browned. Serve with chopped basil or parsley as a garnish. Keep leftovers in the fridge for four days; heat through in the oven preheated to 375°F. You can also freeze leftovers for up to three months.

18. Baked Salmon Pasta

This recipe for salmon pasta is packed with flavor! For a tasty and quick dinner, toss the vegetables and salmon together.

Ingredients

- 1 pint of cut-in-half cherry tomatoes
- 1 box of pasta
- 1 large, finely sliced shallot
- 1 pound of salmon fillets
- 1 tablespoon of drained capers
- 1 tablespoon of olive oil for drizzling
- black pepper freshly ground
- kosher salt
- 1 cup crumbled feta cheese
- 2 teaspoons dried oregano
- 3 tablespoons lemon juice

Instructions

1. Preheat the oven to 425°F. While preparing the vegetables, leave the fish at room temperature. Garnish with chopped fresh Italian parsley or fresh dill. Chop the shallot, garlic, and tomatoes, as previously stated.

2. Add chopped vegetables and drained capers to a 9 x 13-inch baking dish halfway. Join 1 tablespoon olive oil, salt, and newly ground dark pepper in a blending bowl. If it is not already crumbled, add the feta cheese to the skillet in rough chunks and gently stir to combine.

3. The fish should be towel-dried. Divide the filets in half and add a tablespoon of olive oil and 12 teaspoons of kosher salt. To taste, sprinkle with black pepper and dried oregano. Sprinkle with lemon juice after placing the fillets on top of the vegetables in the baking dish.

4. Bake for about 25 minutes. For extremely thin fillets, check at 15 minutes or until the fish is flaky and the internal temperature with a food thermometer is at least 250°F.

5. Bring a pot of salted water to a boil in the meantime. Cook until the pasta is still somewhat firm, then channel. Return to the pan and stir a drizzle of olive oil to prevent sticking.

6. When the salmon is done, transfer it to a plate. Flake it into chunks with a fork.

7. Empty the pasta into the baking dish with the veggies and ¼ teaspoon of salt. Mix in the fish until very much joined. Serve immediately. The remaining food can be stored for two days.

19. Soup with Carrots

This soup with carrots is creamy and colorful! It can be made quickly and has a strong, rich flavor.

Ingredients

- 1 tablespoon fresh ginger, peeled and grated (optional)
- 1 yellow onion
- 3 cloves of garlic
- 1 cup chopped carrots (13/4 pounds, or approximately 12 large carrots)
- 2 tablespoons of olive oil
- 1/4 teaspoon dried dill
- 1/2 teaspoon kosher salt
- 1/4 cup heavy cream
- fresh parsley
- croquettes, to be served (optional).
- Peeling and chopping are required for carrots
- Garlic ought to be minced.

Instructions

1. Sauté the onion for 5 minutes with a little oil. After incorporating the garlic, cook for 1 more minute.

2. Bring the salt, dill, carrots, and vegetable broth to a boil. The carrots should be soft when they are simmered for about 20 minutes.

3. Transfer the hot soup carefully to a blender with a ladle. Add the cream and blend until smooth. Then, add salt, pepper, fresh parsley, and a dollop of cream.

20. Celery Soup

This creamy celery soup is made with a simple recipe! Its fresh flavor and vibrant green color make a statement at any meal.

Ingredients

- 3 teaspoons melted butter (or olive oil)
- 8 ribs finely sliced celery (2 pounds or 4 cups sliced)
- 1/2 medium coarsely sliced yellow onion
- 3 cloves garlic
- 2 medium yellow peeled and chopped potatoes (14 ounces)
- 3/4 teaspoon kosher salt
- 4 cups vegetable broth
- 1/4 tsp dried dill
- 12 cups loosely packed Italian parsley leaves, plus extra for

Instructions

1. In a medium pot, melt the butter over medium heat. Cook for 6 minutes and mix every 2 minutes.
2. Carry to a stew with the hacked potato, vegetable stock, and genuine salt. Cook for 12-15 minutes or until the potatoes are delicate.
3. Transfer the hot soup carefully to a blender with a ladle. Add the parsley and dill and blend. Add the heavy cream and . Serve.

---

21. Mushroom Galette

This substantial mushroom galette recipe is a savory tart loaded with flavor!

Ingredients

- 1/2 cup flour
- 1/4 teaspoon baking powder
- 3/4 teaspoon kosher salt
- 10 tbsp. of kosher salt unsalted virus spread
- 5-6 tablespoons cool water
- 1 egg (for egg wash)
- 4 oz. of cleaned and sliced cremini mushrooms for the filling shiitake mushrooms,
- 2 tablespoons olive oil
- 1 teaspoon garlic powder
- 1 teaspoon soy sauce (or tamari)
- 1 teaspoon dried thyme and smoked paprika
- 1 cup ricotta (whole milk)
- 1 cup Parmesan cheese,

Instructions

1. Mix the flour, a pinch of kosher salt, and baking powder in a bowl. Add onion powder, smoked paprika, thyme, kosher salt, and sprinkle on top the ricotta, Parmesan, garlic, black pepper, and freshly ground sprigs of fresh thyme for garnish. Using a fork, cut the butter and mix it to the flour mixture until it has a pebbly texture (with pea-sized or smaller pieces).
2. Add four tablespoons of cool water to the flour and mix until the water is absorbed. Knead the dough with your fingertips until it comes together by adding an additional 1 to 2 tablespoons of water until all the flour has been added. Don't

add any more water. It ought to work together!

3. Make a thick disk by flattening the dough, transfer the dough to a closed container, and chill for one hour. To make ahead, refrigerate the batter for as long as 3 days; before rolling, allow it to reach room temperature for 30 minutes. If you need to freeze the dough, you have to wrap it in aluminum foil. Defrost overnight in the refrigerator before rolling.

4. The oven should be at 400 degrees Fahrenheit.

5. The mushrooms ought to be cleaned and cut. In a bowl, mix them with soy sauce, olive oil, onion powder, garlic powder, smoked paprika, thyme, and 1/2 teaspoon kosher salt. Bake for about 18-20 minutes in a single layer on a baking sheet lined with parchment paper.

6. Combine the ricotta, Parmesan, garlic, 14 teaspoons of kosher salt, and black pepper in a mixing bowl.

7. Roll the dough into a 12-inch circle on a floured surface, leaving the edges rough. If necessary, move the dough around and add a little more flour underneath to prevent it from sticking. Line a baking with a parchment sheet, and transfer into the dough.

8. Place the mushrooms on top of the dough, gently spreading the ricotta mixture over it. Leave at least 2 inches of dough around the edge. To create a 2-inch crust, fold the dough's outside edges over the filling, overlapping the folds as shown in the images. Use fresh thyme leaves as a garnish.

9. Using a pastry brush, whisk the egg and apply it to the crust. The crust should then be topped with a small amount of flaky sea salt.

10. Bake for about 253 min on a baking sheet. The parchment paper should cool on a baking rack. Let it cool for at least 10 min. It tastes great cold, but you can keep leftovers in the refrigerator for up to three days. Before serving, warm in the oven or bring to room temperature.

22.   Potato Soup

Ingredients

- 3 tablespoons seasoned butter (or olive oil)
- 2 large or 4 small white and light green leeks (4 cups thinly sliced)
- 3 celery ribs
- 3 minced garlic cloves
- 2 pounds peeled and diced russet potatoes (5 cups diced)
- 4 cups vegetable broth
- 1 cup water
- fresh thyme sprigs (or make a bouquet garni)
- 1 bay leaf
- 1 tablespoon kosher salt
- 1/2 cup thick cream.

Instructions

1. Stirring frequently, cook the celery, garlic, and leeks for about 8 minutes: the leeks will become very soft but not browned.
2. Bring the water, salt, chopped potato, vegetable broth, fresh thyme, and bay leaf to a boil. The potatoes should be simmered for 20 minutes or until they are soft. Take out the thyme and bay leaf.
3. Blend everything together and add more cream. Finally, season with salt and pepper.

---

23. Sweet Coconut Raspberry Pancakes

Ingredients

- 2 tbsp flax seed powder + 6 tbsp water
- ½ cup coconut milk
- ¼ cup fresh raspberries, mashed
- ½ cup oat flour
- 1 tsp baking soda
- A pinch salt
- 1 tbsp coconut sugar
- 2 tbsp pure date syrup
- ½ tsp cinnamon powder
- 2 tbsp unsweetened coconut flakes
- 2 tsp plant butter
- Fresh raspberries for garnishing

Directions

1. Mix the flax seed powder with the water in a medium bowl, and allow thickening for 5 minutes.
2. Mix in the coconut milk and raspberries.
3. Add the oat flour, baking soda, salt, coconut sugar, date syrup, and cinnamon powder. Fold in the coconut flakes until well combined.
4. Working in batches, melt a quarter of the butter in a non-stick skillet and add ¼ cup of the batter. Cook until set beneath and golden brown, 2 minutes. Flip the pancake and cook on the other side until set and golden brown, 2 minutes. Transfer to a plate and make the remaining pancakes using the rest of the ingredients in the same proportions.
5. Garnish the pancakes with some raspberries, and serve warm!

---

24. Smoked Tempeh with Broccoli Fritters

Ingredients

For the Flax Egg:
- 4 Tbsp. flax seed powder
- 12 Tbsp. water

For the Grilled Tempeh:
- 3 Tbsp. olive oil
- 1 Tbsp. soy sauce
- 3 Tbsp. fresh lime juice
- 1 Tbsp. grated ginger
- Salt and cayenne pepper to taste
- 10 oz. tempeh slices

For the Broccoli Fritters:

- 2 cups rice broccoli
- 8 oz. tofu cheese
- 3 Tbsp. plain flour
- ½ tsp. onion powder
- 1 tsp. salt
- ¼ tsp. freshly ground black pepper
- 4¼ oz. vegan butter

For serving:
- ½ cup mixed salad greens
- 1 cup vegan mayonnaise
- ½ lemon, juiced

Directions

For the Smoked Tempeh:
1. Mix the water with flaxseed powder in a bowl and soak it for 5 minutes.
2. In another bowl, combine the olive oil, soy sauce, lime juice, grated ginger, salt, and cayenne pepper. Brush the tempeh slices with the mixture.
3. Over medium heat, heat a grill pan and grill the tempeh on both sides until nicely smoked and golden brown, 8 minutes. Transfer to a plate and set aside in a warmer for serving.
4. Mix the broccoli rice, tofu cheese, flour, onion, salt, and black pepper in a medium bowl. Mix in the flax egg until they are well combined and form 1- inch thick patties out of the mixture.
5. Melt the vegan butter in a medium skillet over medium heat and fry the patties on both sides until golden brown, 8 minutes. Remove the fritters onto a plate and set them aside.
6. In a small bowl, mix the vegan mayonnaise with lemon juice.
7. Divide the smoked tempeh and broccoli fritters onto serving plates, add the salad greens, and serve vegan mayonnaise sauce.

25. Herbed Seafood Casserole Preparation

Ingredients

- ½ c. uncooked long-grain rice
- 2 tbsp. unsalted butter
- 1 medium onion, finely chopped
- 3 celery ribs, thinly sliced
- 1 medium carrot, shredded
- 2 Garlic cloves, minced
- ¼ tsp. Pepper · ½ tsp. salt
- ½ Tbsp. minced fresh parsley
- 1 ½ tsp. Snipped fresh dill or ½ tsp. dill weed

For the Seafood:
- 1 ¼ lb. uncooked shrimp
- 1 lb. bay scallops
- 1 can crab meat
- 1 ½ c. half-and-half cream
- 5 tbsp. unsalted butter, cubed
- ¼ c. all-purpose flour
- ½ tsp. Snipped fresh dill or ½ tsp. dill weed
- 1 package (8 oz.) low-fat cream cheese
- ½ tsp. Salt
- ¼ tsp. Pepper
- ¼ tsp. dried thyme

For the Toppings:
- ½ Tbsp. butter, melted
- 1 ½ c. soft breadcrumbs

Directions

1. Preheat the oven to 325°F. Cook rice according to package directions. In the meantime, in a big skillet, heat butter over moderate heat. Add onion, celery, garlic, carrot, salt, and pepper. Cook for about 5 minutes or until crisp-tender. Combine with the cooked rice and add parsley and dill. Put in a baking dish.
2. Fill a large saucepan with ⅔ full of water and bring to a boil. Include shrimp (peeled and deveined) and simmer for about 40-45 seconds. Add scallops; simmer for 3 minutes or until shrimp turn pink and the scallops are firm and dense. Reserve 1 cup of cooking liquid. Put the seafood in a large bowl; stir in crab meat (drained, flaked, and cartilage removed).
3. Melt the butter in a pan. Stir in flour until mixed; slowly stir in cream and keep cooking liquid. Boil within 2 minutes or until condensed and foamy. Add the cream cheese cubed and dill. Cook over medium heat for a few minutes. Stir into the seafood blend.
4. Pour over the rice mixture. Sprinkle over the top of the buttered breadcrumbs. Bake, uncovered, for 50 minutes or until it turns golden brown. Stand 10 minutes before dishing.

26. Turkey Medallions

Ingredients

- 20 oz. turkey tenderloins, sliced
- 1 egg
- 3 tbsp. olive oil
- 2 tbsp. lemon juice
- 1 c. panko breadcrumbs
- ½ c. Parmesan cheese, grated
- ½ c. walnuts, chopped
- 1 tsp. Lemon-pepper seasoning
- ¼ tsp. pepper
- fresh basil, chopped

Directions

1. Mix egg and lemon juice in a bowl.
2. Mix breadcrumbs, nuts, lemon pepper seasoning, and cheese in a separate bowl.
3. Season turkey with pepper.
4. Preheat oil in a skillet over medium heat.
5. Dip each turkey piece first into the egg mixture and the breadcrumb mixture. Add to the skillet and cook for 2-3 minutes per side. Serve topped with basil.

27. Italian Stuffed Artichokes

Ingredients

- 4 large artichokes
- 2 tsp. lemon juice
- 2 cups soft Italian breadcrumbs, toasted

- ½ cup grated Parmigiano-Reggiano cheese
- ½ cup minced fresh parsley
- 2 tsp. Italian seasoning
- 1 tsp. grated lemon peel
- ½ tsp. pepper
- ¼ tsp. salt
- 1 Tbsp. olive oil

Directions

1. Level the bottom of each artichoke using a sharp knife and trim off 1-inch from the tops. Snip off the tips of outer leaves using kitchen scissors, then brush lemon juice on the cut edges. In a Dutch oven, stand the artichokes, pour 1-inch of water, and then boil. Lower the heat, put the cover, and let it simmer for 5 minutes or until the leaves near the middle pull out effortlessly.
2. Turn the artichokes upside down to the drain. Allow it to stand for 10 minutes. Carefully scrape out the fuzzy middle part of the artichokes using a spoon and get rid of it.
3. Mix the salt, pepper, lemon peel, Italian seasoning, garlic, parsley, cheese, and breadcrumbs in a small bowl, add olive oil, and stir well. Gently spread the artichoke leaves apart, then fill them with the breadcrumb mixture.
4. Now spray an 11x7-inch baking dish with cooking spray and place artichokes. Let it bake for 10 minutes at 350 °F without cover or until the filling turns light brown.

2-Week Meal Plan

WEEK 1			
D	**BREAKFAST**	**LUNCH**	**SNACK P.M.**	**DINNER**
1	Challah French toast	Quick Hummus and Turkey Medallions	Cheese Balls	Wraps of Lasagna and Fruit Dip in a Flash
2	Oatmeal Baked with Pumpkin	Wraps of Lasagna	Pumpkin chocolate chip bread	Quick Hummus and Turkey Medallions
3	Cranberry orange muffins	Pumpkin French Toast and Italian Stuffed Artichokes	Cheese Balls	Potato Soup and Fruit Dip in a Flash
4	Challah French toast	Mediterranean Tuna Salad	French Toast Sticks	Pumpkin French Toast and Italian Stuffed Artichokes
5	Oatmeal Baked with Pumpkin	Mediterranean Tuna Salad	Fruit Dip in a Flash	Potato Soup and Fruit Dip in a Flash
6	Cranberry orange muffins	Pumpkin French Toast	Cheese Balls	Herbed Seafood Casserole Preparation
7	Sweet Coconut Raspberry Pancakes	Celery Soup and Italian Stuffed Artichokes	Fruit Dip in a Flash	Mushroom Galette and Delicious Sweet Potato Bites

WEEK 2			
D	BREAKFAST	LUNCH	SNACK P.M.	DINNER
8	Sweet Coconut Raspberry Pancakes	Mushroom Galette and Quick Hummus	Delicious Sweet Potato Bites	Baked Salmon Pasta
9	Breakfast Bowls with Cottage Cheese	Baked Salmon Pasta	French Toast Sticks	Mushroom Galette and Quick Hummus
10	French Toast Sticks	Smoked Tempeh with Broccoli Fritters	Delicious Sweet Potato Bites	Soup with Carrots and Cheese Balls
11	Pumpkin chocolate chip bread	Kale Barley Salad and Italian Stuffed Artichokes	Cheese Balls	Mushroom Galette and Quick Hummus
12	Breakfast Bowls with Cottage Cheese	Kale Barley Salad	French Toast Sticks	Soup with Carrots and Turkey Medallions
13	French Toast Sticks	Celery Soup and Turkey Medallions	Pumpkin chocolate chip bread	Herbed Seafood Casserole Preparation
14	Pumpkin chocolate chip bread	Celery Soup and Italian Stuffed Artichokes	Pumpkin chocolate chip bread	Mushroom Galette and Delicious Sweet Potato Bites

BONUS: VIDEO PLAYLIST

With you in mind, I have created a playlist in which introductory and other videos on the vague nerve are grouped.

Subscribe to the channel and enjoy !!!

Conclusion

A solid eating routine is significant for ideal vagus nerve well-being. A diet high in fruits, vegetables, whole grains, and lean proteins can aid in digestion and reduce inflammation. Additionally, reducing the consumption of sugar and processed foods can contribute to improved overall health.

A healthy diet and getting enough vitamins and minerals are important. B vitamins, magnesium, and zinc, among other vitamins and minerals, have been shown to reduce inflammation and improve nerve health. It's also important to drink enough water.

It is possible to improve nerve health and reduce inflammation by drinking a lot of water. Lastly, getting enough sleep is essential for the health of the vagus nerve. Stress can be lessened, and overall health can be improved by getting 7-8 hours of sleep each night.

There are several supplements that can help improve the health of the vagus nerve, in addition to eating a healthy diet and getting enough sleep. Inflammation can be reduced, and nerve health can be improved with these supplements. Omega-3 fatty acids are one supplement that can help improve nerve health. Omega-3 fatty acids can improve nerve health and reduce inflammation.

Magnesium is another supplement that can help maintain healthy nerves. Magnesium has been shown to improve nerve health and reduce inflammation.

Additionally, a vital supplement for nerve health is vitamin B complex. Inflammation can be reduced, and nerve health can be improved with vitamin B complex. Lastly, zinc is an essential supplement for healthy nerves. Zinc can aid in nerve health and inflammation reduction.

Because it is a vital nerve in the body, activating the vagus nerve can help improve overall health. Yoga, deep breathing, humming, gargling, and other exercises can stimulate the vagus nerve.

For optimal vagus nerve health, it's also essential to get enough sleep and eat well. Lastly, several supplements can help improve nerve health and reduce inflammation.

That's all there is to it! Thanks to this guide, you should now be able to harness the power of your vagus nerve and improve your overall health. Keep yourself healthy and safe!

References

1.(https://www.forbes.com/sites/womensmedia/2021/04/15/what-the-vagus-nerve-is-and-how-to-stimulate-it-for-better-mental-health/?sh=65f240b76250)

2.(https://www.getsensate.com/blogs/news/everything-vagus-nerve)

3.https://www.insider.com/guides/health/mental-health/vagus-nerve-exercises

4.https://www.mindbodygreen.com/articles/should-you-be-toning-your-vagus-nerve-heres-how-to-hit-the-reset-button

5.https://www.goodnet.org/articles/try-these-exercises-that-activate-vagus-nerve

6.https://www.parsleyhealth.com/blog/how-to-stimulate-vagus-nerve-exercises/

7.https://www.arcvic.org.au/34-resources/402-vagus-nerve-exercises

8.https://health.clevelandclinic.org/vagus-nerve-stimulation/

9.https://mentalhealthmatch.com/articles/anxiety/4-vagus-nerve-exercises-for-anxiety

10.https://www.sportskeeda.com/health-and-fitness/vagus-nerve-exercises-that-will-rewire-your-brain

11.https://themovementparadigm.com/tag/vagus-nerve-stimulation-exercises/

12.https://bebrainfit.com/vagus-nerve-stimulate/

13.https://health.howstuffworks.com/wellness/diet-fitness/exercise-at-work/10-office-exercises-you-can-do-secretly.htm

14.https://chopra.com/articles/a-yoga-practice-to-activate-the-vagus-nerve

15.https://www.yogauonline.com/yoga-practice-tips-and-inspiration/6-ways-stimulate-your-vagus-nerve-yoga-and-breathing

16.https://healthnews.com/family-health/healthy-living/vagus-nerve-massage-does-it-work/

17.https://www.parsleyhealth.com/blog/how-to-stimulate-vagus-nerve-exercises/

18.https://drruscio.com/vagus-nerve-diet/

19.https://bodybio.com/blogs/blog/how-to-stimulate-vagus-nerve

20.https://www.ndtv.com/health/these-simple-and-effective-exercises-can-help-melt-belly-fat-within-no-time-do-include-them-in-your-1970403

21.https://www.flintrehab.com/stroke-exercises/

22.https://www.healthline.com/health/migraine/stretches-for-migraine#side-neck-bend

23.https://omronhealthcare.com/blog/home-remedies-and-healthy-habits-for-neck-and-shoulder-pain/

24.https://health.usnews.com/conditions/respiratory-disease/bronchitis/articles/exercising-with-bronchitis-what-you-should-know

25.https://www.somnologymd.com/2017/03/exercise-for-insomnia/

26.https://www.healthline.com/health/ten-best-menopause-activities#yoga-and-meditation

27.https://www.acouplecooks.com/category/recipes/

28.https://www.acouplecooks.com/category/recipes/breakfast-brunch-recipes/

29.https://www.acouplecooks.com/gluten-free-lunch-ideas/

30.https://www.acouplecooks.com/category/recipes/?_search_recipes=lunch

31.https://www.acouplecooks.com/category/recipes/everyday-healthy-dinner-recipes/

32.https://www.acouplecooks.com/category/recipes/appetizers-healthy-snack-recipes/

Made in United States
Orlando, FL
06 May 2023

32868713R00059